The Ultimate
Fast Metabolism Diet
Cookbook

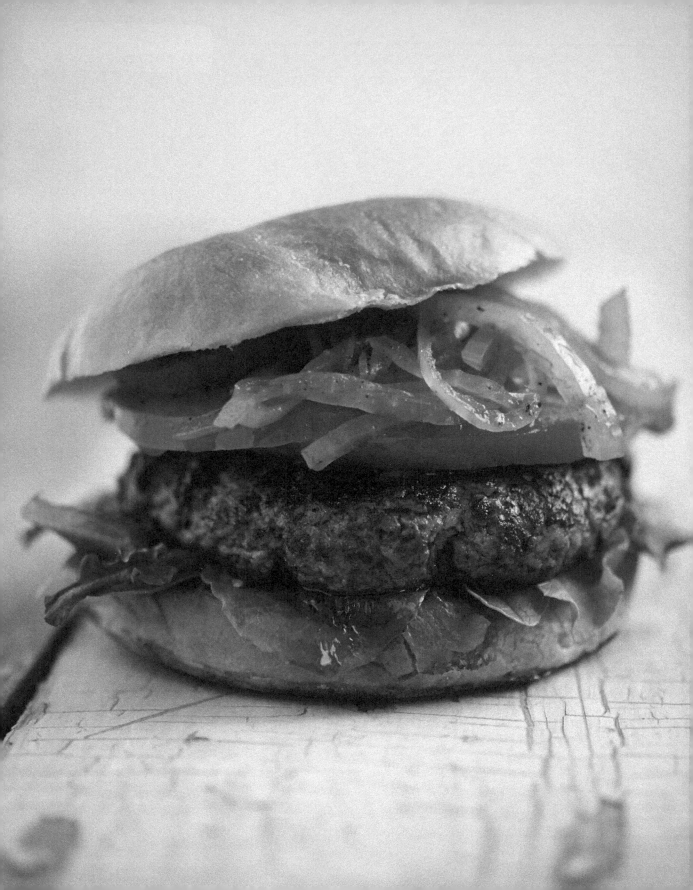

The Ultimate Fast Metabolism Diet Cookbook

Quick and Simple Recipes to Boost Your Metabolism and Lose Weight

ROCKRIDGE
PRESS

Quick Start Guide

Ready to jumpstart your metabolism right away? *The Ultimate Fast Metabolism Diet Cookbook* has everything you need. Just follow these six steps:

1 Understand what affects your metabolism and its relationship to weight loss. See page 15.

2 Familiarize yourself with the diet's three stages: Repair, Release, and Reignite. See page 21.

3 Adopt an exercise program. See page 24.

4 Stock your kitchen and pantry with all the foods and ingredients you need for each of the three stages. See page 32.

5 Stay focused and on track with a wealth of recipe options. See page 46.

6 Propel yourself forward with your new lifestyle.

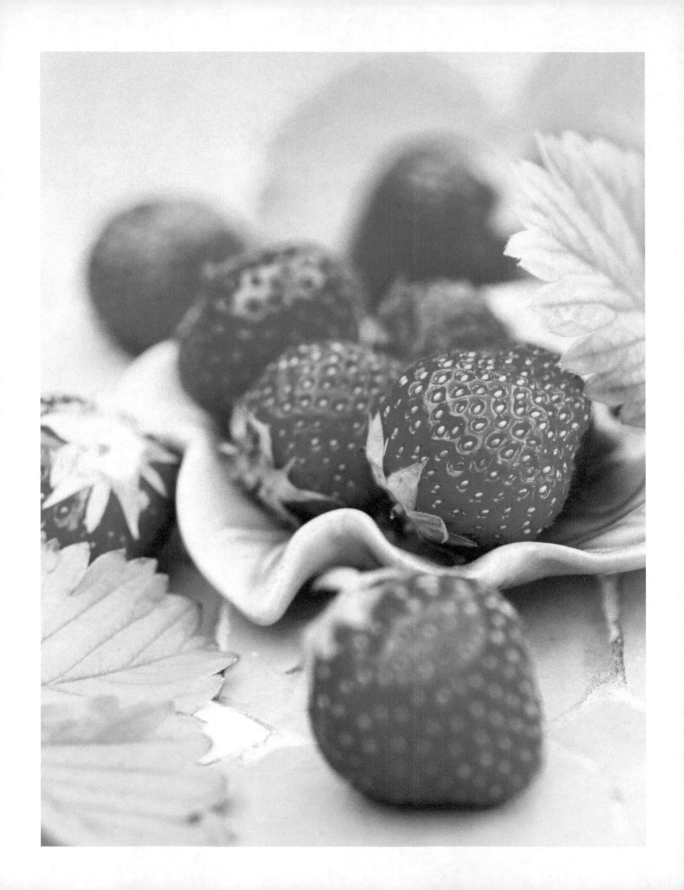

Contents

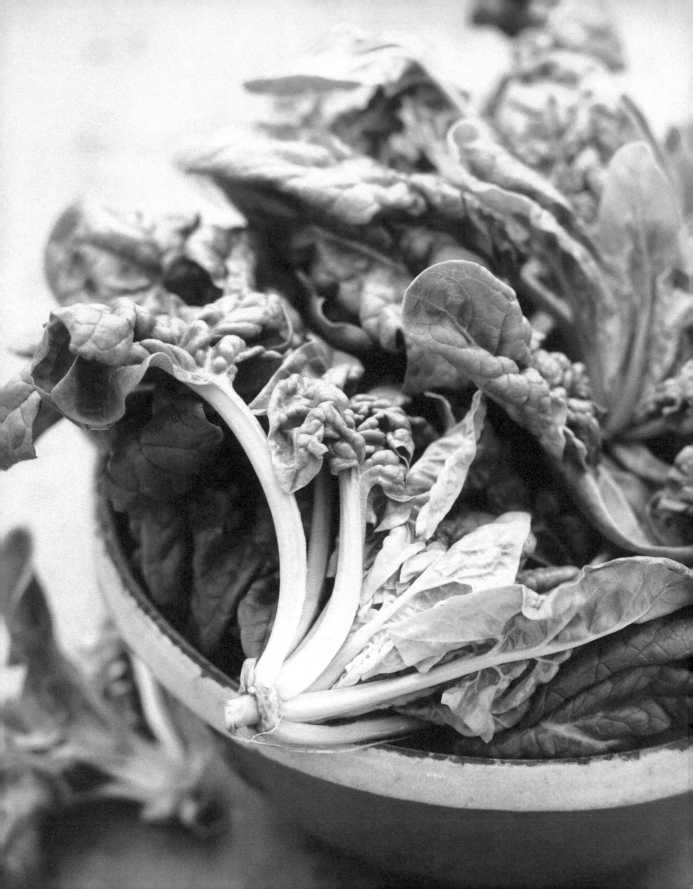

Introduction

If you're following the Fast Metabolism Diet, there's a good chance that, like so many people, you've discovered your metabolism has slowed down over the years. Most of us simply can't eat anything and everything the way we used to without gaining weight.

The Fast Metabolism Diet is a great way to reboot your metabolism. By removing highly processed, chemical-laden foods and focusing on meals made from whole, natural ingredients, prepared in your own kitchen, you can help your body recover from years of eating the kinds of foods that have made your metabolism more sluggish than you'd like it to be. Best of all, and unlike most diets, you are actually required to eat—five times a day, and sometimes more.

If you're already on the Fast Metabolism Diet, you know the principles behind it are not particularly complicated. But it can be difficult to adapt the diet to everyday life, especially if you're not used to doing a lot of cooking.

The Ultimate Fast Metabolism Diet Cookbook is here to give you more options as you eat your way to a slimmer you. You'll find over 200 great-tasting, wholesome meals, snacks, and desserts that are satisfying and easy to prepare. This book also offers meal-planning tips that set you up for success by showing you how to follow the diet and shop for essential pantry and refrigerator items, as well as a sample 28-day meal plan.

In Part One, we'll review how to eat to boost your metabolism for weight loss in just 28 days. We'll look at the basic principles of the Fast Metabolism Diet, and outline the three-stage approach to jumpstart your metabolism.

Part Two of this book features over 200 recipes—more than you'll find anywhere else for the Fast Metabolism Diet. They include classic American dishes, nourishing comfort foods, and international favorites. With recipes for breakfast, lunch, dinner, snacks, and even desserts, you won't feel deprived. All the recipes feature healthy whole foods that have been shown to enhance your metabolism.

Everyone is busy these days, and it's difficult enough to find time to prepare meals for your family, let alone make a separate "diet" meal for yourself. That's why the recipes in this book have been developed with your entire household in mind. With hundreds of recipes to choose from, all of which simply taste like good food, you're sure to find family favorites at every stage of the diet for every meal.

The recipes in this book are here to help you eat deliciously through all 28 days of the Fast Metabolism Diet. Many will become favorites that you return to again and again, helping you sustain your healthy new lifestyle beyond the initial four-week program. They are easy to cook and don't require exotic ingredients or a long series of complicated steps and techniques. Most can be prepared in under an hour; some have a longer cooking time, but you need not tend them while they bake or simmer in the slow cooker.

Your small investment in time and effort will have a big payoff in flavor, health, and weight loss. You'll be preparing whole, healthy, unprocessed foods that not only boost your metabolism, but also taste great and are deeply satisfying.

Part One

GETTING STARTED

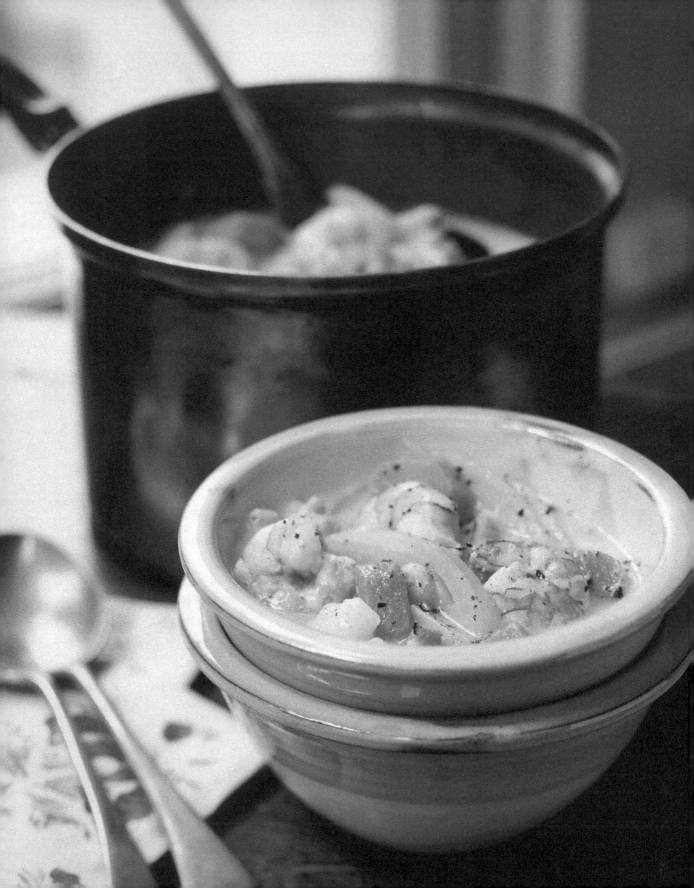

Chapter One

Fundamentals of the Fast Metabolism Diet

Whether you're new to the Fast Metabolism Diet or are already on the diet and picked up this book for the 200-plus recipes, it's important to go over its principles. Many authors and dietitians have developed diets to boost metabolism. These plans rely on similar principles to detoxify your body and kick your metabolism into higher gear. The information in this chapter will review the basics of these diets and how and why this program can work for you.

Your first step is to take a closer look at the main attraction: your metabolism. What is it exactly? How does it function? And most important, what does it have to do with your weight? Understanding the answers to these questions will help you make lifelong smart food choices.

What Is Metabolism?

At its simplest, metabolism is a chemical process that occurs in your body that helps it sustain life. When we're taking about diet specifically, it's a process by which your body uses energy from food to complete its basic biological processes and sustain the activities of daily living.

Everything your body does burns energy. Many of these body processes are automatic, such as breathing. In fact, a majority of the food energy (commonly referred to as calories) you burn—about 60 to 75 percent—goes to fuel these basic bodily functions, which include:

- Respiration
- Circulation
- Cell growth
- Immune function

The remaining 25 to 40 percent of the energy your body burns fuels two specific areas:

- Physical movement
- Eating, digestion, and elimination

Some people have a metabolism that is very efficient. That is, the body uses only small amounts of food energy to carry out biological tasks. People with an efficient metabolism are said to have a "slow" metabolism, because their bodies do not require very much food energy to sustain the activities of daily living.

Your metabolism plays a significant role in determining how you gain, lose, or maintain your weight. While many people believe weight gain or loss is a simple equation of calories in versus calories burned, individual variations in metabolism can make that equation very complicated. That's why one person can eat 3,000 calories per day and not gain weight, while someone else may struggle to lose weight eating 1,200 calories per day.

For years, eating less and moving more has been the standard advice for weight loss (or avoiding weight gain). And it is true that if you can create a caloric deficit—regularly burning more calories than you eat—you will lose weight. However, how many calories a person needs to function varies widely,

Factors That Affect Metabolism

Metabolism varies greatly from person to person because it is influenced by so many factors.

- **Lean body mass:** According to the Colorado State University fact sheet "Nutrition and Aging", metabolism decreases as lean body mass decreases. Lean body mass is everything in your body that is not fat, including muscles, organ tissue, and bone. Therefore, maintaining or building muscle mass can have a positive effect on metabolism.

- **Insulin levels:** Insulin plays an important role in the body, signaling cells to convert blood sugar (glucose) into energy. However, as Gary Taubes explains in his book *Good Calories, Bad Calories*, the amount of insulin circulating in the bloodstream affects what your body does with that glucose. When insulin levels are high, insulin acts as a fat-storage hormone, causing your body to store calories as fat instead of using it as fuel.

- **Activity levels:** The more you move, the more fuel your body requires. Some studies show that people who constantly fidget burn food energy more quickly. Likewise, the positive effects of exercise and movement on weight loss are well documented by medical literature.

- **Stress levels:** Recent medical literature points to high or chronic stress levels as strongly correlating with weight gain and obesity. Researchers believe this may be related to the release of the hormones epinephrine and cortisol during stress, which reduce insulin sensitivity.

- **Sleep deprivation:** Sleep—or lack thereof—has a profound effect on your metabolism. This effect may occur for a number of reasons, including changes in levels of the hormones ghrelin and leptin, which control hunger, according to WebMD. Chronic sleep deprivation is also a stressor, which affects levels of cortisol and epinephrine.

- **Food:** The types of food you eat certainly affect your metabolism. For example, processed foods contain chemicals that may affect hormone levels, while sugar and starch affect insulin levels.

- **Medications:** Some prescription and over-the-counter medications may affect your metabolism. Check with your doctor about the medications you take and any effect they may have on your metabolism.

depending on one's metabolism. Two people of the same age, sex, height, weight, and activity level may have very different metabolic requirements.

People with a more sluggish metabolism may find they tend to gain weight even when they're on restrictive diets and get plenty of exercise, while people with a faster metabolism may be able to maintain a more sedentary, higher-calorie lifestyle without gaining weight. For those on the slower end of the metabolic spectrum, this can feel quite frustrating.

Principles of a Fast Metabolism Diet

Several different versions of a fast metabolism diet are available today, written by authors such as Jillian Michaels, Dr. Michael Mosley, and Haylie Pomroy, but they all have many common principles that make up the basis of the rec-ommendations for a fast metabolism eating program. The recipes in this book are based on these common principles. Keep these principles in mind as you pursue your Fast Metabolism Diet.

Eliminate highly processed foods. Basically, that means avoid anything that comes in a bag, box, or package and has a long list of unpronounceable ingredients. A good general rule is this: If your great-grandparents wouldn't recognize it as food, you probably shouldn't eat it. This includes foods like nutrition bars, protein powders, crackers, potato chips, and many others. These contain all sorts of ingredients that can jam up the works of your metabolism. If you must buy packaged foods, read the labels carefully to ensure they don't contain any of the ingredients you specifically should not eat on the Fast Metabolism Diet.

Also eliminate foods that are commonly derived from genetically modified organisms (GMOs) such as soy and wheat, as well as industrial seed oils, which are refined in an industrial process. Replace oils and fats like shortening, mar-garine, canola oil, sunflower oil, soybean oil, or corn oil with extra-virgin olive oil, which is far less refined and contains beneficial monounsaturated fats.

Eliminate artificial enhancers and sweeteners, caffeine, and alcohol. That includes the sweeteners aspartame, sucralose, acesulfame potassium (acesulfame K), and saccharine. Avoid foods that contain artificial colorings and dyes, preservatives, and artificial flavorings. Also avoid caffeine, soda (diet soda, too!), coffee, alcoholic beverages, and similar foods and drinks that don't support good health.

Eliminate empty calories. To supply your body with the vitamins and minerals it needs, it is essential to eat nutrient-dense foods that pack plenty of vitamins and minerals into every calorie. To that end, cut out all foods that are high in calories but don't have much nutritional value. This includes sugar, high-fructose corn syrup, candy, and very starchy grains like wheat and corn.

Eliminate gluten and dairy. According to Haylie Pomroy's *The Fast Metabolism Diet*, many people are sensitive to these foods, while others have difficulty processing the proteins they contain. Even for people who aren't sensitive to them, however, gluten and dairy can cause inflammation and gut irritation, which can slow metabolism. To the best of your ability, remove gluten and dairy from your diet. You'll find gluten in anything that contains wheat, barley, or rye, such as most baked goods. You'll also find it hidden in foods that may surprise you, such as mustard and soy sauce. Read labels carefully. Avoiding dairy includes eliminating butter, cheese, milk, ice cream, yogurt, whey, casein, lactose, and similar products and ingredients.

Focus on real, whole foods. Choose simple, whole, nutritious foods that are as close to the source from which they came as possible. Select fresh fruits

The Macronutrients

Foods contain two types of nutrients essential for life: macronutrients and micronutrients. Micronutrients include vitamins and minerals, while macronutrients include protein, fat, and carbohydrates.

Proteins are made up of amino acids and include animal foods such as meat, fish, poultry, and eggs. Complete plant food proteins include foods like tofu and edamame, seitan, and tempeh. You can also create complete plant proteins by combining foods such as rice and beans.

Carbohydrates are sugars, fibers, and starches that elevate blood glucose levels. Different types of carbs elevate blood glucose to different extents. In general, simple sugars create a rapid elevation in blood glucose, while complex carbohydrates cause a more gradual rise. Meats contain virtually no carbohydrates. However, you'll find carbs in all products that contain grains, as well as in fruits, vegetables, nuts, seeds, legumes, tubers, dairy products, candy, baked goods, and many other food items. Natural sugars like honey and pure maple syrup also contain carbohydrates.

and vegetables, healthy whole grains, nuts and seeds, and fresh meat and eggs. For example, choose a whole chicken as opposed to a mechanically separated, breaded, fried chicken nugget; or eat a baked sweet potato instead of French fries cooked in industrial seed oils.

Confuse your metabolism. Avoid sticking to any particular eating "style" for more than a few days. The Fast Metabolism Diet calls for you to cycle through three stages every week. This keeps your body from adapting to the diet—which would cause it to burn calories more efficiently and slow your metabolism. Some plans achieve metabolic confusion by fasting or varying the caloric intake significantly each day. This program achieves metabolic confusion by cycling through variations of macronutrient levels, including carbohydrates, protein, and fat. By alternating among high-glycemic low-fat, low-carb low-fat, and low-glycemic moderate-fat meals, you'll keep your metabolism from adapting to any specific macronutrient profile.

The Week-Long Three-Stage Approach

The recipes in this book are meant to work as part of a four-week (28-day) Fast Metabolism Diet. Four weeks gives you enough time to completely reboot your metabolism. During that time, you will cycle each week through three stages. Each stage has a specific purpose, and cycling through the three stages creates metabolic confusion.

This three-stage approach works for several reasons.

- Each stage offers a specific macronutrient profile that helps you control your blood sugar. Rapid rises in blood sugar trigger large amounts of insulin in the bloodstream. As we mentioned, insulin in excess causes the body to store fat. Rapid rises and falls in blood sugar are associated with food cravings and sensations of hunger. The three-stage approach allows you to maintain consistent hunger levels and avoid cravings.

- The three stages ease you into eating whole, real foods that support good health. They also help you eliminate chemical-laden foods that can harm your health and slow your metabolism. Over the course of the four weeks, your body will detoxify from the toxic content of the standard American diet.

- Each stage offers micronutrients, macronutrients, and healthy fats your body needs for good health. According to the USDA, the best way to get all the vitamins and minerals your body needs is to eat foods in a rainbow of colors. The three stages cycle you through foods with different micronutrient profiles, ensuring that your body receives a full complement of vitamins and minerals.

- Each stage is short. That way, you're only in the most restrictive stages for two days at a time. This short duration makes it easier to get through the restrictive stages, with more choices coming soon.

THE RULES

As with every eating plan, the Fast Metabolism Diet has a few definite dos and don'ts. These rules will help ensure your success, so it's important to follow them.

- Do check with your doctor. Talk to your health care professional before starting any new diet or exercise program.

- Do eat three meals and two snacks every day. Because the foods are calorie controlled, it is important to eat every few hours to provide your body with the energy it needs to support bodily functions and avoid blood sugar crashes or cravings.

- Do control your portions. Since calories are a consideration, it's important to limit yourself to the portion sizes noted in the recipes.

- Do drink plenty of water. The diet calls for you to give up other beverages, including juice, coffee, and soda, making water even more important. Not only will water help you flush the toxins from your body, but it also will keep you hydrated and can help you feel satiated.

- Do follow the recipes as they are written. Don't make substitutions unless there is one noted for the recipe.

- Do plan ahead. Create a menu plan each week, listing which meals you'll have in each stage. From there, make a shopping list and shop only for the items on your list. A four-week meal plan is included in this book, if you'd prefer to follow it.

- Do set up your environment for success. Remove tempting off-plan foods from your pantry, cupboards, and refrigerator. Instead, stock up on the healthy foods you'll need to be successful.

- Do exercise. Exercise is an essential part of good health. If you're currently very sedentary, start with walking around your neighborhood and work your way up to more strenuous exercise. Make sure you include stretching in your exercise routine.

- Do minimize stress. Even when you're eating healthy foods, stress can change your hormone profiles. Minimize stress and find ways to cope with it, such as exercise, yoga, or meditation.

- Do get plenty of sleep. Sleep deprivation can change hormone levels, slowing your metabolism.

- Do allow yourself plenty of time at the grocery store. If you buy food in cans, jars, bags, and boxes, read the ingredients carefully.

- Do make the diet as easy as possible for yourself. If you have particularly busy weeknights, make meals on the weekends and store them to eat during the week.

- Do wait for a craving to pass. Cravings may seem intense, but they often pass quickly. Instead of giving in to a craving, distract yourself with some other activity until it passes.

- Do set goals. Set obtainable goals for yourself each week, such as making time to exercise or following the diet exactly, and then reward yourself with nonfood items such as a warm bath or an early bedtime.

- Don't skip breakfast. While many people miss this important meal, you'll need it to provide yourself with enough energy to get through the day. Studies show that people who skip breakfast end up feeling hungrier and eating more during the day. Eating breakfast will also help control cravings.

- Don't get down on yourself if you slip up. Sometimes even the most dedicated dieters have a slip. If you do, simply get back on the plan as quickly as possible.

The Three Stages: Repair, Release, Reignite

The Ultimate Fast Metabolism Diet Cookbook offers recipes that cycle through three stages:

Repair—fix the damage to your system

Release—access the energy trapped in your body

Reignite—get your body to burn calories and fat at a faster rate

Each week, you will follow Stage One for two consecutive days, Stage Two for two consecutive days, and Stage Three for the remaining three consecutive days of the week. The stages will cycle you through meals and snacks with different macronutrient profiles.

STAGE ONE: REPAIR (MONDAY–TUESDAY)

During this stage, you will eat foods designed to support your body as it begins the process of detoxification. The meals in this stage will also begin to heal damage caused by the standard American diet. Along with getting rid of toxic ingredients, Repair stage foods encourage hormonal balance by providing adrenal support. As you replace processed foods from the standard American diet with nourishing, whole foods, you will begin to flush out the toxins that have built up over the years.

How to Eat

In the Repair stage, the foods you prepare and eat will be:

- Sugar-free, caffeine-free, alcohol-free, chemical-free, gluten-free, dairy-free, artificial sweetener-free.

- Filled with high-glycemic fruits, vegetables, and whole grains to help you get past initial cravings from the removal of sugar and junk foods, while providing you with energy as your body transitions from the standard American diet to a new way of eating.

- Moderate in lean protein to support lean tissue and help avoid hunger, without causing undue stress on the body related to excess protein consumption.

- Low in fat, so that the foods you eat are rich in vitamins and minerals.
- Moderate in calories to help avoid hunger.
- Nutrient-dense with vitamins and minerals, such as vitamins B, C, and antioxidants, that assist your detoxification and raise energy levels.

How to Exercise

In the Repair stage, be gentle on your body as you initiate its repair.

- Pursue low- to moderate-intensity activity such as walking, low-impact or nonimpact aerobic exercise (such as swimming or the elliptical trainer), yoga, light calisthenics, and stretching.
- Stretch before and after every exercise session.
- Warm up for five minutes before every exercise session with gradually increasing intensity.
- Cool down for five minutes by gradually decreasing intensity.

Stage One Food List

This stage emphasizes high-vitamin, high-energy, high-glycemic-index foods, such as:

- Fruits like apples, cherries, plums, citrus fruits, pears, bananas, mangos, and pineapples.
- Root vegetables and tubers such as potatoes, sweet potatoes, onions, rutabagas, and carrots.
- Leafy greens like spinach, kale, and lettuce.

The glycemic index is a measure of how quickly your blood sugar rises when you eat a certain food. *All foods with carbohydrates are rated based on how they affect your blood sugar. The glycemic index (GI) assigns a number from 0 to 100, showing how quickly your blood sugar rises when you eat that food. The scale is based on a piece of white bread, which causes blood glucose to spike quickly and has a glycemic index of 100. High-glycemic-index foods have a GI number of 51 or above, while low-glycemic-index foods have a number of 50 or below.*

- Cruciferous vegetables like cabbage, cauliflower, and broccoli.
- Whole grains like quinoa, rice, and gluten-free whole grain pasta.
- Lean proteins such as white meat chicken, white meat turkey, egg whites, fish, shellfish, mollusks, and extra-lean beef.
- Legumes such as chickpeas, lentils, black beans, white beans, and kidney beans.
- Healthy fats—mostly extra-virgin olive oil.
- Natural sweeteners, including honey, stevia, and pure maple syrup.
- Herbs and spices.

STAGE TWO: RELEASE (WEDNESDAY–THURSDAY)

During the Release stage, the goal is for your body to release energy that has been stored (primarily as fat). In this stage, carbohydrate intake is lowered significantly in order to reduce insulin release. Without excess amounts of insulin circulating freely in your blood, your fat cells will dispense the energy that has been stored there. This stage improves the way your body releases insulin into the bloodstream in the presence of glucose, so it optimizes your body's use of food as energy.

At the same time, this stage is high in nutrient-dense vegetables, particularly low-carb veggies. The nutrients in these vegetables help you continue to detoxify while supporting your body's energy needs.

How to Eat

In this stage, you will:

- Continue avoiding sugar, caffeine, alcohol, fruit juice, soda, chemicals, artificial sweeteners, and processed foods.
- Eat a moderate amount of lean animal protein, such as egg whites, chicken breast, turkey breast, fish, and extra-lean beef.
- Eat plenty of low-carbohydrate, non-starchy vegetables, such as dark leafy greens, mushrooms, bell peppers, broccoli, and zucchini.
- Keep carbohydrate intake at 50 grams per day or less, all from vegetables.
- Eat a small amount of nuts and seeds.

- Avoid or minimize starchy vegetables such as potatoes, carrots, and sweet potatoes.
- Avoid or minimize fruit intake to limit sugar and carbohydrates.
- Avoid natural sweeteners like honey or maple syrup (stevia is fine).
- Avoid all grains.

How to Exercise

While this stage is fairly restrictive because it is low in fat and low in carbohydrates, you will still have plenty of energy to exercise. In fact, exercising will help you further release stored fat. The release of stored fat into the blood will give you the energy you need for exercise.

- Do moderate- to high-intensity strength training. All the protein you're eating during this stage helps you rebuild muscle fibers broken down by strength training. Lift weights to muscle exhaustion, in three sets of 8 to 10 repetitions, to build strength.
- Focus on large muscle groups. Exercises that work the large muscle groups will also exercise smaller muscle groups. For example, the bench press primarily works your chest, but your triceps, shoulders, and forearms also get a workout as you lift. Squats work your gluteal muscles, but they also work quadriceps, hamstrings, and calf muscles.
- Balance muscle groups. If you work your chest and shoulder muscles, be sure to work your back muscles as well. If you work your quadriceps, work your hamstrings. If you work your biceps, work your triceps as well. When you work your abs, also work your lower back.
- Don't do strength training that works the same muscle group two days in a row. Your body needs time between sessions for repair, so allow at least 48 hours or more.
- Warm up with light activity on the muscle groups you will be working.
- Cool down with low-intensity activity to allow your blood to return from your extremities to your core.
- Stretch every muscle you have worked before and after the workout.

Stage Two Food List

During this stage, the list of foods you can eat will be restricted to the following:

- Lean proteins like chicken breast, turkey breast, fish, shellfish, egg whites, and lean meats.
- Leafy greens like spinach, kale, Swiss chard, arugula, and lettuce.
- Non-starchy vegetables like zucchini, broccoli, radishes, and celery.
- Very low-glycemic-index fruits, like tomatoes.
- Nuts and seeds in very limited amounts because of the fat content.
- Extra-virgin coconut oil in limited amounts.
- Extra-virgin olive oil in limited amounts.
- Herbs and spices.
- Stevia.

STAGE THREE: REIGNITE (FRIDAY–SUNDAY)

This stage is designed to really rev up your brand-new metabolism. While you continue eating whole, naturally healthy foods that are full of vitamins, you'll add high-energy foods that your body can use for fuel. With low-glycemic-index carbs in the mix, you'll also keep your blood glucose and insulin levels steady so your body will still have access to the stored energy (in the form of fat) you released in the previous stage. You'll add a little more fat too, particularly healthy fats containing omega-3 fatty acids, which will help decrease inflammation and provide an extra boost of energy.

What to Eat

In this stage, you will:

- Continue to stay away from all of the toxic foods you've been avoiding so far, like caffeine, chemicals, gluten, GMO soy, and dairy.
- Eat lots of healthy low-glycemic-index vegetables.
- Eat a moderate amount of healthy low-glycemic-index fruits like berries, tomatoes, and cantaloupe.

- Eat occasional low-glycemic-index grains, such as quinoa, millet, or brown rice.
- Eat moderate amounts of protein, including occasional consumption of higher fat proteins from time to time.
- Eat plenty of coldwater fish high in omega-3 fatty acids.
- Eat a moderate amount of nuts and seeds that contain healthy fats.
- Eat low-glycemic-index legumes occasionally.
- Eat a moderate amount of healthy fats including coconut oil and extra-virgin olive oil.
- Eat natural sweeteners like maple syrup and honey very occasionally.

How to Exercise

Since you're firing up your metabolism, this is a great time to do one of the best types of metabolism-boosting exercises: high-intensity interval training (HIIT). You can do HIIT on any piece of aerobic equipment, or while riding a bicycle, walking, or jogging. To perform HIIT:

- Warm up with five minutes of gradually increasing intensity.
- Do very high-intensity activity for one minute. To do this, pedal faster, sprint, or set a steep incline on your treadmill.
- Do low-intensity activity for three minutes. Jog lightly, walk, take a leisurely pedal, or walk along a flat incline.
- Repeat the cycle of high intensity and low intensity four to seven more times.
- Cool down with five minutes of gradually decreasing intensity.
- Stretch.

Stage Three Food List

During this stage, you will be much less restricted than you were before. You can eat:

- Low-glycemic-index fruits like avocados, tomatoes, berries, cantaloupe, and honeydew, as well as a small amount of juice from lemons and limes.
- Low-glycemic-index vegetables like cauliflower, celery, fennel, green beans, asparagus, artichokes, cabbage, onions, broccoli, sweet bell peppers, chili peppers, summer and winter squash, jicama, and mushrooms.

- Low-glycemic-index root vegetables like carrots, parsnips, celery root, turnips, and sweet potatoes.

- Dark leafy greens such as Swiss chard, kale, lettuce, arugula, and spinach.

- Animal proteins like fish, shellfish, mollusks, beef, pork, lamb, game meats, and eggs.

- Legumes like black beans, white beans, kidney beans, chickpeas, cashews, and peanuts.

- Low-glycemic-index grains like brown rice, amaranth, and quinoa.

- Nuts and seeds like almonds, pecans, chia, pumpkin seeds, walnuts, and sesame seeds.

- Pure natural sweeteners like stevia, organic honey, and pure maple syrup.

- Healthy fats like extra-virgin olive oil and extra-virgin coconut oil.

- Herbs and spices.

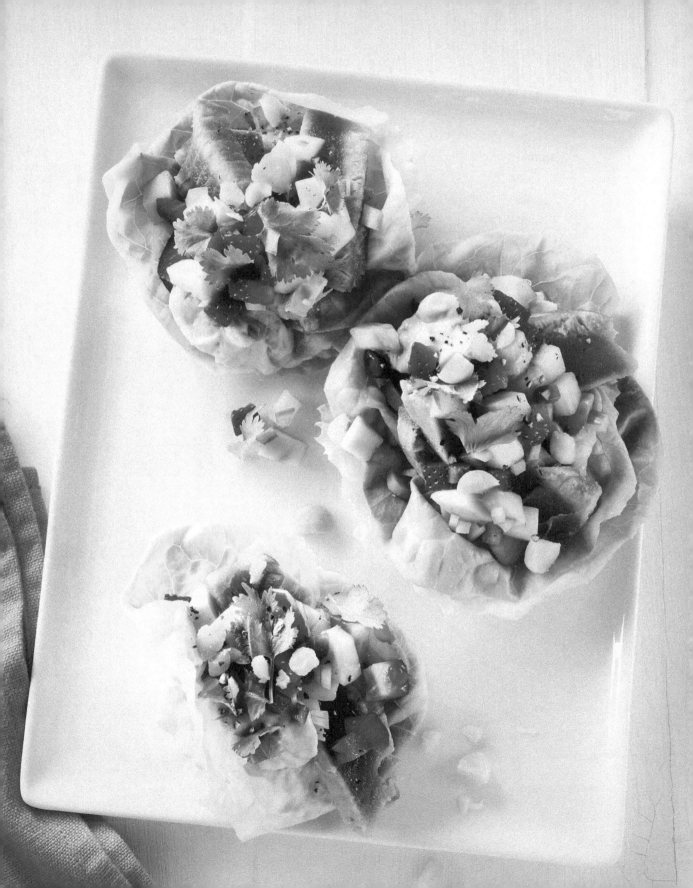

Chapter Two

How to Use *The Ultimate Fast Metabolism Diet Cookbook*

The more than 200 recipes in this book are great for even the most novice chef. Not only do they incorporate a variety of delicious flavors and cuisines, but most of them also have short lists of ingredients, and many can be whipped up in less than 15 minutes. Along the way, you will gain tips and insights on how to save prep and cooking time, how to stock your pantry, and how to shop smarter and save money to make your four-week commitment to the Fast Metabolism Diet as stress-free as possible.

The recipes highlight the main foods and ingredients for each stage so you know what you are eating and how it relates to your metabolism. You can, therefore, create a stronger bond between your new diet and your goal of boosting your metabolism and losing weight.

Tips and Tricks for Success

From shopping and food preparation to adjusting to a new way of eating, you are bound to face obstacles as you adjust to this diet program. Here are some tips for making your journey as smooth as possible.

- Be realistic. People grow frustrated with diets because they set the bar too high. If you begin this diet thinking that you'll lose 30 pounds in a month, you're setting yourself up for failure. Instead, focus on the short-term goal of eating to fire up your metabolism. As you improve your metabolism every day, you will soon begin to notice the pounds and inches melting away.

- Celebrate your successes. Your body is just beginning the process of improving your metabolism. Don't fill your head with self-doubt and memories of previous diet failures. Instead of focusing only on weight loss, stay in the present and constantly remind yourself that you've already made a great accomplishment—you've made the first move to boost your metabolism. Celebrate the beginning of your journey, and eventually, you will celebrate the achievement of your goals.

- Keep a journal. A journal, or even a blog, can keep you motivated and increase your ability to lose weight. A 2008 study published in the *American Journal of Preventive Medicine* found that those who kept a food journal could double their diet weight loss. Your journal/blog acts as a personal support group and cheering section to help you deal with the highs and lows of a diet. At the end of each day, write down your thoughts and feelings about your progress, what you liked, what felt good, and what you struggled with.

- Change your dishes. A common complaint about most diet plans is that they make you feel deprived. If your servings seem skimpy, change your perspective. Use smaller plates to give the impression that you are eating more food. You are less likely to feel "cheated" if the entire plate surface is covered.

COOKING FOR MORE THAN ONE

- Buy in season. Check your newspaper's food or cooking section for information about in-season produce, which is often less expensive. You can also shop at your local farmers' market for great deals; prices may be lower because there are fewer transportation costs.

- **Go generic.** Store brands are cheaper than big brand names and often contain the exact same ingredients. However, compare labels to ensure that you get the same product. Ingredients are listed in order by weight, so canned tomatoes, for example, should have tomatoes listed first, and not water.

- **Sold out? Get a rain check.** When popular items go on sale, they tend to sell out quickly. That doesn't mean you're out of luck. Ask about getting a rain check, so you can pick up the item later at the sale price. If the store runs out of sale items, they're supposed to offer a rain check—but you have to ask for it.

- **Buy in bulk.** Some items, like meats, rice, and beans, can be purchased in bulk to save money. You may also want to think about joining a warehouse shopping club like BJ's, Sam's, or Costco for additional savings.

- **Listen to your own music when you shop.** Ever wonder why grocery store music is soft and relaxing? It encourages you to shop more slowly and ultimately buy more food. To speed up your shopping, put in your earplugs and listen to a favorite workout mix or upbeat tunes instead.

- **Can the canned beans.** Cooking up a bag of dried beans is much less expensive than buying them in cans. It's not time-consuming or hard to do, and a bigger batch means you are less likely to run out. Canned beans sometimes have added salt. Also, bagged beans create less waste than canned beans, so your garbage can will fill up more slowly. However, if you don't have time to make a pot of beans, then by all means buy them in cans so you can save time when you cook.

- **Skip the cut-up fruits and vegetables.** If it gets sliced up and packaged, it costs more. Buy your fruits and veggies whole and cut them up yourself, unless you're in a hurry and would otherwise skip the produce; in that case, consider precut fruits and veggies as the time-savers they are.

————————

This book has recipes that the entire family can enjoy. Have everyone sample the recipes and, when you find meals they enjoy, you can make double portions and freeze them for later family meals.

————————

You Can Freeze Meat for About Six Months. *Divide large cuts of meat into meal-size portions and wrap each portion in freezer paper. Wrap carefully, so every millimeter of the meat is covered. Write the contents and date on the wrapper. Store the portion-size packages in your freezer in heavy-duty, zip-top freezer bags. This way, you can defrost only what you need.*

- Buy larger portions of meat. It's cheaper to buy big portions than individual cuts. Ask the butcher to cut up larger roasts into small portions for you.

- Pack lunches and snacks the night before. Lunch can often be problematic, since you usually eat it away from home. Preparing your lunch each day right before you leave for work or school can be stressful, and you might even forget it in the rush of your morning routine. Instead, try to make your lunch the night before, perhaps when you are making dinner, so you can just grab it and go in the morning.

- Keep snacks on hand. Don't get caught without your twice-a-day snacks. Make a batch of snacks from the recipes, and keep them handy for easy access—at home, in the office, and on the go. This will help block any temptations to reach for vending-machine foods or other unhealthy choices.

- Make meals special. When you eat, focus on your food and nothing else. Unplug from the TV, put away your work, and shut down your computer. The more distracted you are, the faster you tend to eat, and the less likely you will feel full and satisfied. Slow down. Take the time to chew so you enjoy the simple act of savoring food. A study in the *Journal of the American Dietetic Association* found that people reported greater satiety when they ate slowly, rather than rushing through their meals.

Stocking Your Kitchen

Setting up your kitchen to begin cooking for the Fast Metabolism Diet is quite straightforward. There are a few foods that you will be banning completely from your daily meals, including wheat (most breads, crackers, and pastas), dairy products (butter, yogurt, and cow's milk), refined white sugar, caffeine, and alcohol. If at all possible, remove these items from your pantry and refrigerator shelves so you aren't tempted to cheat, and replace them with foods that will help you achieve success while you are healing your metabolism.

Here is a list of the foods you'll want to keep on hand as you cycle through the recipes in this book.

REFRIGERATOR/FREEZER

Dairy Substitutes and Eggs

- Cultured yogurt made from almond milk or coconut milk: These nondairy products are great stand-ins for dairy-based yogurt. You can use them interchangeably. Buy plain, unsweetened, unflavored versions of these products.

- Nondairy milk: Many of the recipes in this book call for rice milk, coconut milk, or almond milk. Choose plain, unsweetened varieties. Opt for rice milk during the Repair stage, and then switch to coconut or almond milk for the Release and Reignite stages of the diet.

- Eggs: Eggs are a staple throughout all three stages of the diet. If you can, buy fresh eggs from locally raised chickens. These eggs are much fresher and more flavorful than the ones in the grocery store.

Meat, Poultry, and Seafood

- Beef: Select lean cuts of beef, such as skirt steak. If you can find it, choose grass-fed beef, which is lower in fat and higher in omega-3 fatty acids.

- Ground meats: In the Repair and Release stages of this diet, the focus is on low-fat foods, so you will want to stock low-fat ground meats such as ground turkey or chicken breast, and extra-lean ground beef or bison. In the Reignite stage, you can eat fattier meats such as ground pork, ground veal, ground lamb, and higher-fat ground beef. If you can find it, choose meat from naturally pastured (grass-fed) animals; grass-fed meat is lower in fat and higher in healthy omega-3 fatty acids than its grain-fed counterparts.

- Deli-sliced meats: Deli chicken, turkey, ham, and roast beef are perfect for a quick snack. Select gluten-free versions that don't contain sugar.

- Pork: In the Repair and Release stages, choose pork tenderloin, which is very lean. In the Reignite stage, you can add other cuts of pork, such as pork chops or occasional servings of bacon.

- Poultry: In the Repair and Release stages, choose very lean poultry, such as boneless, skinless chicken or turkey breasts. In the Reignite stage, you can enjoy slightly fattier cuts such as skin-on thighs.

- Fish and seafood: Purchase fresh or frozen seafood, including wild-caught salmon, halibut, trout, shrimp, and scallops. You can also keep a few cans of water-packed tuna on hand for a quick snack.

Fresh Produce

- Bell peppers and chiles: These ingredients add flavor and crunch to many dishes. Stock jalapeños, red bell peppers, green bell peppers, and any other peppers that appeal to your palate.

- Berries: Berries are low-glycemic-index, low-carb options for all stages of this diet. They make great snacks and side dishes. Stock blueberries, strawberries, raspberries, cranberries, and blackberries.

- Carrots and celery: These make great low-carb snacks. When paired with onions, carrots and celery also form a threesome revered in most cuisines that serves as an aromatic flavor base for many recipes.

- Citrus fruits: The recipes here make liberal use of fresh citrus juice and zest to add flavor and brightness to recipes. Keep lemons, limes, and oranges on hand.

- Flaxseed: Flaxseed contains beneficial omega-3 fatty acids, which are especially important during the Reignite stage. Because they are high in these volatile fats, the seeds must be refrigerated.

- Herbs: Fresh herbs bring vibrancy and flavor to many of the recipes here. Keep fresh herbs such as rosemary, oregano, parsley, cilantro, dill, basil, tarragon, and chives on hand. Pick a few of your favorites—you don't

---

Vegetarian or Vegan? No Problem. *When meat is required in a recipe, you can often switch it out for another protein source, like legumes, beans, or eggs. Or you can simply stick with the recipes marked vegetarian or vegan.*

---

need them all. With the exception of basil, everything can be stored in the refrigerator. Keep basil at room temperature in a vase with a little bit of water.

- **Leafy greens:** Dark leafy greens contain fiber and antioxidants necessary for good health. The recipes in this book call for several types of dark leafy greens, including kale, Swiss chard, spinach, collard greens, and lettuce.

- **Melons:** Many melons (with the exception of watermelon) are low in carbs and have a low glycemic index, so they make great snacks. Stock cantaloupe and honeydew.

- **Onions and garlic:** These two aromatic vegetables form the flavor base for many of the recipes here. Keep onions, red onions, and garlic cloves in your pantry, and keep scallions in the refrigerator.

Frozen Produce

- **Frozen herbs in olive oil:** A simple way to stretch your food budget is to freeze leftover chopped fresh herbs using an ice cube tray. Spoon one tablespoon of herbs into each cube section, and then cover with olive oil. You can use these frozen oil-and-herb blocks in place of fresh herbs and oil in any recipe.

- **Frozen fruits and vegetables:** Keeping frozen fruits and vegetables in your freezer gives you a shortcut for many of the recipes that follow. These precut items will save you lots of prep time when you are in a hurry.

PANTRY

- **Agar powder:** This vegan alternative to gelatin is made from red algae and is used in recipes to gel, thicken, and stabilize ingredients. It's flavorless and high in protein and fiber.

- **Arrowroot powder:** Arrowroot is a starchy, protein-rich root vegetable widely grown in the Philippines, Caribbean islands, and South America. In its powder form, it's often used as a gluten-free alternative to cornstarch or flour as a thickening agent for sauces, puddings, and fillings. Arrowroot powder is used in all stages of the Fast Metabolism Diet.

- **Broth:** Many recipes call for chicken or vegetable broth. Choose low-sodium, gluten-free options for your pantry.

- **Legumes:** Legumes such as chickpeas, white beans, black beans, lentils, and kidney beans are staples of the Fast Metabolism Diet. Keep a variety of dried and canned legumes to use in the recipes here. Read the labels and make sure there's no added salt.

- **Canned tomatoes:** Keep a variety of canned tomato products in your pantry, including tomato paste, crushed tomatoes, and whole tomatoes. Choose brands that don't contain sugar, artificial chemicals, or synthetic sweeteners.

- **Cocoa powder:** Unsweetened cocoa powder is used in recipes for all three stages of the Fast Metabolism Diet, from smoothies to shakes and pudding.

- **Coffee (decaffeinated):** Though your morning cup may be banned, you'll be happy to know that you can still enjoy the flavor of coffee in some of your meals. Keep a small container of decaf ground coffee in the pantry.

- **Condiments:** Select gluten-free, sugar-free condiments, such as soy sauce, fish sauce, Dijon mustard, coarse-ground mustard, tahini, Worcestershire sauce, and sugar-free sriracha sauce. Commercial mayonnaise often contains high-fructose corn syrup and sugar, but it's actually very easy to make your own (see page 37).

- **Gluten-free bread and flour:** A few recipes in this book call for gluten-free bread. Choose whole-grain sandwich bread, and keep it in the refrigerator if you won't eat it all in a few days. If the bread goes stale, simply process it in the food processor or blender to create bread crumbs, which you can keep in a zip-top bag in the freezer. A few recipes also call for gluten-free flour, which can be found in the specialty aisle of most grocery stores.

- **Gluten-free grains:** Though the Repair stage of the program does allow high-glycemic grains such as brown rice, the Reignite stage calls for only low-glycemic-index grains such as quinoa, oats, and millet.

- **Honey:** Unlike refined sugar, which has no nutritional benefits, this natural sweetener is packed with antioxidants.

- **Liquid smoke:** Just a drop or two of this condensed liquid will add a smoky flavor that reminds you of bacon and other fatty barbecue staples—without the added fat. If you cannot find liquid smoke or do not like its intensity, try substituting smoked paprika or chipotle powder.

Make Your Own Condiments

Most commercially processed condiments are full of unnecessary added sugars or high-fructose corn syrup. But it's actually quite easy to make your own healthy versions of these classic condiments in your own kitchen. Give these go-to recipes for homemade sriracha and mayonnaise a shot and continue to enjoy the flavors of some of your favorites.

Do-It-Yourself Sriracha

Most sriracha sauce is loaded with sugar. Read the label very carefully to find a sugar-free brand, or make it yourself.

12 ounces red jalapeño peppers, with seeds, stemmed and sliced
8 garlic cloves, chopped
1 teaspoon sea salt
1½ cups apple cider vinegar
1 packet stevia

1. In a large, sterilized mason jar, combine the jalapeños, garlic, salt, and apple cider vinegar. Screw on the lid and shake the jar to mix up all of the ingredients.

2. Leave the jar to sit at room temperature overnight.

3. After 12 to 24 hours, transfer the contents of the jar to a medium saucepan and heat on medium-high heat until it simmers. Add the stevia. Reduce the heat to low and simmer for 5 minutes. Cool to room temperature.

4. In a blender purée the cooled mixture until it is smooth. Store in a sterilized mason jar in the refrigerator. It will keep for up to 1 month refrigerated.

Easy Homemade Mayonnaise

Eliminate the sugar and high-fructose corn syrup found in commercial processed mayonnaise by making your own Easy Homemade Mayonnaise. You can make flavored mayonnaise by adding a minced garlic clove, a dash of chipotle powder, chopped herbs, or some lemon or lime zest. This mayonnaise keeps well in the refrigerator for up to five days.

1 egg yolk
1 tablespoon red wine vinegar
½ teaspoon Dijon mustard
¼ teaspoon fine sea salt
¼ teaspoon freshly ground black pepper
¾ cup olive oil

1. In a food processor or blender, combine the egg yolk, red wine vinegar, mustard, salt, and pepper. Process to combine the ingredients.

2. With the food processor or blender running continuously, begin to add the oil through the chute or opening in the lid. Add the oil one drop at a time to start, until you've added about 20 drops of oil. Then continue adding the oil in a very thin stream until the mayonnaise has completely emulsified.

- Nonstick cooking spray: It's great for greasing skillets and pans while reducing the amount of oil you need to cook.

- Nuts and seeds: In the Reignite stage, you will eat healthy fats, and nuts and seeds are excellent sources. Stock your pantry with nuts like walnuts and cashews, as well as sugar-free nut butters such as peanut butter and almond butter. You can also enjoy seeds such as sunflower, sesame, and pumpkin seeds.

- Oil: You will need a variety of oils to make the recipes in this book. The most commonly used are light and extra-virgin olive oils, but some recipes also call for sesame oil, walnut oil, and extra-virgin coconut oil.

- Salsa: Jarred salsa makes an excellent snack, as well as a good topping for meat or eggs. You can use jarred salsa throughout all stages of the diet, as long as it doesn't contain any legumes, corn, or sugar.

- Stevia: Stevia is a natural sweetener that doesn't affect your blood sugar and is used in some of the recipes in this book. You can purchase stevia in many forms, including liquid and powder. Different brands of stevia have varying levels of sweetness, so you may need to adjust the amount you use depending on the brand you purchase.

- Tea (decaffeinated): Green tea and some herbal teas are full of beneficial nutrients and antioxidants. For this diet, always choose decaffeinated teas; the ones you'll need for the recipes are green, chamomile, and orange pekoe.

- Vinegar: Vinegar brings brightness and acidity to foods throughout all stages of the Fast Metabolism Diet. You can use virtually any type of vinegar, except for malt vinegar, which contains gluten. Stock a variety of vinegars, including red wine vinegar, distilled white vinegar, apple cider vinegar, and balsamic vinegar.

Get Ready Ahead of Time. *Since this diet program requires a firm commitment on your part, make sure your life is ready. Review the recipes for the first week and stock up on everything a few days beforehand. Put major house projects on the back burner. You want to begin when everything is as stress-free as possible, so you can just focus on yourself and the diet.*

Spice Rack

- Black peppercorns: Freshly ground black pepper is more flavorful than preground. You can buy whole peppercorns in the spice aisle of the grocery store and then grind them yourself in an inexpensive pepper grinder.

- Dried herbs: Dried herbs substitute well for fresh herbs in a pinch. Keep dried herbs such as basil, coriander, oregano, tarragon, Italian seasoning, marjoram, thyme, savory, and rosemary in your spice rack.

- Garlic and onion powder: Keep these two spices on hand. They add flavor quickly when you don't have time to chop and sauté onions and garlic.

- Salt: Most of the recipes here that include salt call for sea salt. Choose a fine-grained sea salt, which works well in all recipes. You may also want to have kosher salt in the pantry, which is exceptionally good for seasoning meat before cooking.

- Spices: Both sweet and savory spices are used in many of the recipes in this book. Stock your spice rack with cinnamon, ground nutmeg, ground mace, ground allspice, ground ginger, ground cloves, ground cumin, celery seed, dried mustard, cayenne pepper, paprika (sweet and smoked), chili powder, chipotle powder, and red pepper flakes.

- Spice blends: Some spice blends are used in the recipes that follow; they can be handy because you don't have to create your own. Check to make sure the spice blends don't contain sugars or gluten. Stock Chinese five-spice powder, Old Bay seasoning, and curry blends.

- Vanilla extract: Vanilla extract is great for adding a warm, sweet flavor to recipes without too much added sweetener. It's used for many of the sweet recipes in this book. Buy the best quality vanilla extract you can—many lesser brands contain propylene glycol, artificial flavors, and other adulterants.

ESSENTIAL EQUIPMENT

You don't need a kitchen that is tricked out with all the latest appliances and expensive cookware to make the recipes in this book. In fact, chances are you already have everything you need. Here is a list of kitchen equipment that will help you make the most of the next four weeks on the Fast Metabolism Diet.

Cooking Tools

- Chef's knife: A high-quality knife is essential in every kitchen. A chef's knife is big—usually about eight inches long—with a blade that's wide near the grip and tapers down to a point. It can be used for mincing, slicing, and chopping. Choose one that feels comfortable in your hand and holds a sharp edge.

- Knife sharpener: Keeping your knives sharp improves their safety and functionality. You can choose an electric or a hand sharpener to maintain these important tools.

- Mixing bowls: Use glass or stainless steel mixing bowls in a variety of sizes.

Appliances That Save You Time

There are many pieces of equipment that will help make your job easier. You don't actually need any of these items, but they will save you a great deal of time and effort in the kitchen.

- Blender and/or food processor: These two pieces of equipment save you tons of cutting, chopping, and mixing time in the kitchen, and help you make foods such as mayonnaise, smoothies, and pesto. Even an inexpensive, small-capacity food processor can help you save extra time as you cook. In many cases, you can use an affordable immersion blender (sometimes called a stick blender) in place of these two pieces of equipment.

- Electric mixer or stand mixer: A mixer can save you time while cooking, although it's not necessary. Anything you can do with a mixer, you can also do by hand.

- Microwave oven: While not essential, a microwave is helpful for reheating leftovers and cutting corners on cooking times.

- Slow cooker: Perhaps one of the most popular pieces of time-saving equipment is the slow cooker. With a slow cooker, you can prepare your ingredients in the morning, toss them in the cooker, and come home to a fully cooked dinner. Look for a slow cooker with a large capacity and easy-to-use controls. It's also helpful to have a tight-fitting lid and several temperature settings, including high, low, and warm.

Are Portion Sizes Important?

How much you eat is every bit as important as what you eat. Even the best diets can go awry if portions are too large. You want consistency in how much you eat from day to day, but the individual portions of some foods may vary. For instance, you will notice that the recipes in each of the three stages are not designed around a specific number of calories; rather, your three daily meals and two snacks fall squarely into the range your body needs to support its regular, ongoing functions.

The individual portions for some items change depending on the stage you're in, because you may need more or less of certain nutrients. For instance, in the Repair stage, the primary goal is to detox your metabolic system, so you will consume fruits and vegetables that are high in antioxidants. During the Reignite stage, you'll eat more healthy fats to get your body to burn calories at a faster rate. So while portion sizes are an important part of any diet, you have to think beyond size and look at substance, too.

- Utensils: You'll need the usual array of kitchen utensils, including wooden spoons, a spatula, a carrot peeler, a meat thermometer, a paring knife, a rubber scraper, a large wire whisk, and a set of measuring spoons and measuring cups.

Pots and Pans

- Baking pans: Keep several high-sided metal or glass baking pans. You will need pie pans, 9-inch square pans, and 9-by-13-inch rectangular pans.

- Baking sheet: Have several 10-by-15-inch metal baking sheets.

- Cast iron skillet: A cast iron skillet is a multifunctional tool in the kitchen. It goes easily from stovetop to oven and can cook virtually any food. It also serves as a sauté pan and a nonstick fry pan. Get a 12-inch skillet and keep it well seasoned to maintain the skillet's functionality.

- Dutch oven: A Dutch oven is a heavy pot with a tight-fitting lid that can go from the stovetop to the oven. Use it to make soups and stews. Buy one with ovenproof handles, so you can use it for braising and roasting.

- Saucepans with lids: Keep saucepans in an array of sizes for cooking soups, sauces, and stews, as well as for gently rewarming foods.

Frequently Asked Questions

Q: Do I have to give up alcohol?

A: You don't have to give up your glass of wine or weekend beer forever, but for the next four weeks, you should indeed avoid all alcoholic beverages. In order to detox and boost your metabolism, you have to protect it from outside stress.

Q: I am a vegetarian/vegan. Can I eat soy?

A: Yes, but in limited amounts. Soy foods may affect your thyroid gland, which can slow your metabolism. Your thyroid releases two hormones—triiodothyronine (T3) and thyroxine (T4)—that control metabolism. Some research suggests that soy intake can cause hypothyroidism and disrupt hormone production. In fact, a 2011 study published in the *Journal of Clinical Endocrinology and Metabolism* found that participants experienced a threefold increase in their risk of developing hypothyroidism after consuming 16 milligrams of soy supplement per day over an eight-week period. The science is still inconclusive, but to be on the safe side, the recipes in this book contain little to no soy. A dash or two of gluten-free soy sauce is the only exception.

Q: Can I work the desserts into my meals for the week?

A: Like the rest of the recipes in this book, the desserts have been designed to boost your metabolism. Eat a stage-appropriate dessert as one of your snacks, or have it after dinner and add an extra day of exercise to your weekly routine.

Q: Do I have to eat organic foods?

A: While organic foods, especially fruits and vegetables, are more expensive and debate continues as to whether they are in fact healthier, we recommend that you eat organic whenever possible. Remember, you are trying to restore your metabolism, so you want to reduce your intake of toxins—whether by eliminating processed foods or your exposure to pesticides, insecticides, and hormones. But don't let cost sway you. Think of it as an investment in your health. The money you spend today will pay off with lower weight and better health as you move forward.

Q: Do I have to begin the program on a Monday?

A: No. You can start any day of the week, but many people find it easiest to begin a new dietary program at the beginning of a new week. Do all of your grocery shopping and prepare your ingredients ahead of time, so you're ready to jump in—and stick with it—whenever you choose to start the diet.

Q: How much weight can I expect to lose?

A: That depends on your current weight, body size and composition, and current metabolic health. If you have a lot of weight to lose—twenty or more pounds—you may lose weight at a faster pace once your metabolism is functioning at a high level again. However, don't focus too much on a set number. Instead, work on getting your metabolism healthy. Once you begin to drop pounds, you can set a realistic weight-loss goal.

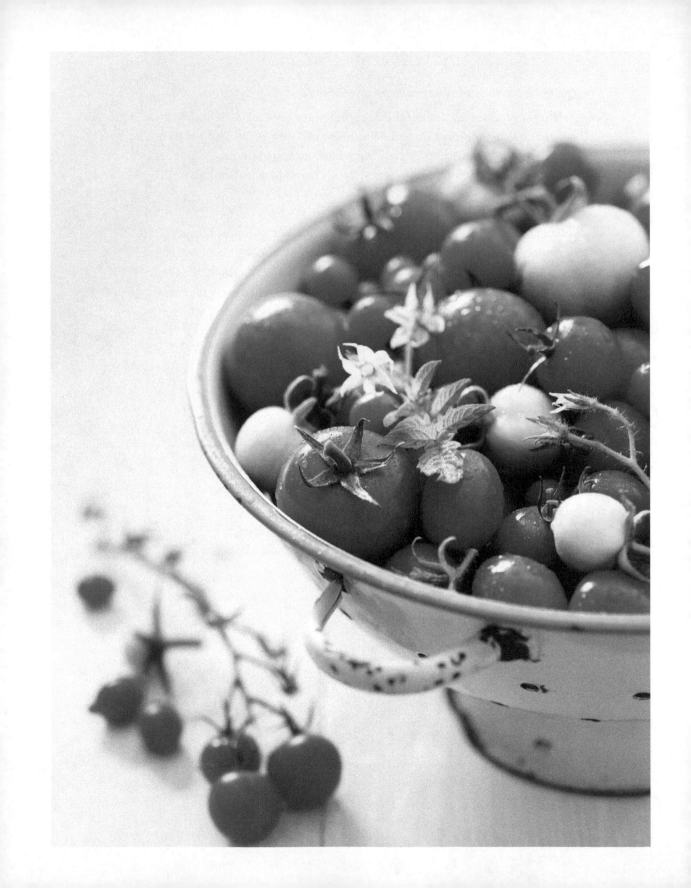

Part Two

THE RECIPES

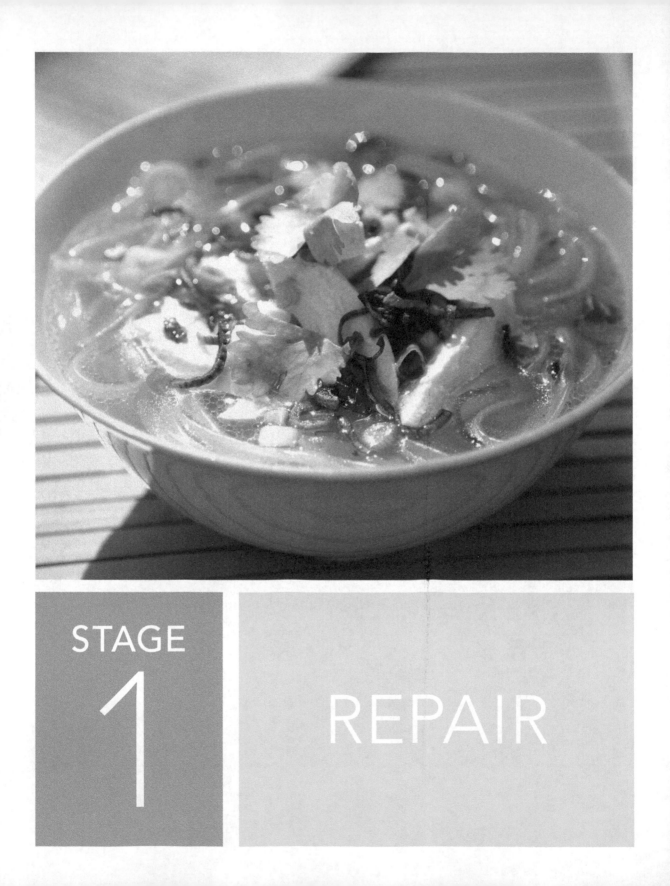

STAGE

1

REPAIR

STAGE 1 RECIPES

Breakfast

Blueberry-Banana Smoothie 49
Green Tea Smoothie 50
Spiced Baked Apples with Flax 51
Apple and Pear "Pie" 52
Coconut Yogurt and Melon Parfait 53
Breakfast Rice 54
Slow Cooker Cranberry-Orange Oatmeal 55
Hot Quinoa Breakfast Cereal with Flax 56
Almond Butter and Banana Toast 57
Pumpkin Pancakes 58
Dutch Apple Pancake 60
French Toast with Warm Berry Compote 61
Sweet Potato Waffles 63

Lunch

Minted Cantaloupe and Cucumber Salad 64
Tomato and Orange Chopped Salad 65
Gingered Peach and Rice Salad 66
Quinoa Salad with Lemon and Peppers 67
Pesto Chicken Pasta Salad 68
Gazpacho 69
Easy Chicken Rice Soup 70
Thai Rice Noodle Soup with Turkey 71
Open-Faced Prosciutto, Fig, and Arugula
    Sandwich 73
Chicken and Grape Salad Sandwich 74
Chicken Breasts with Blackberry Sauce 75
Pork Tenderloin with Mustard and Plums 76

Snacks

Herbal Tea Smoothie 77
Piña Colada Chia Smoothie 78
Chocolate Shake 79
Carrot and Fruit Salad 80
Three-Bean Salad 81
Baked Sweet Potato Crisps 82
Chickpea and Zucchini Hummus 83
Pumpkin Dip 84
Black Bean and Pineapple Salsa with
    Corn Chips 85
Mediterranean White Bean Dip with
    Vegetables 86
Crispy Toasts with Tomato Basil
    Bruschetta 87
Pecan Granola Bars 88

Dinner

Eggplant and Artichoke Casserole 89
Quinoa Pasta with Sautéed Mushrooms 91
Brown Rice Bowl with Vegetables 92
Slow Cooker Wild Rice with Mushrooms and
    Dried Cranberries 93
BBQ Baked Beans and Greens 94
Hearty Potato-Leek Soup 96
Baked Sweet Potato with Pineapple 97
Halibut with Mango and Watercress Salad 98
Baked Red Snapper with Summer Fruit 99
Citrus-Ginger Salmon 100
Cioppino 101
Mussels in Tomato Sauce 103
Baked Scallops with Mango Salsa 104 »

Dessert

Blueberry-Banana Smoothie

SERVES 1 / PREP TIME: 5 MINUTES

Smoothies offer nearly endless possibilities for refreshing breakfasts that won't weigh you down. In this one, the addition of rice makes for an especially thick, rich treat. You can use leftover cooked unseasoned brown or white rice. For an even thicker smoothie, use frozen blueberries instead of fresh.

Time-saving tip: *You don't need to cook the rice yourself if you don't have time. You can buy precooked plain rice from the freezer or rice section at the grocery store to use in smoothies and other dishes.*

1 navel orange, peeled and sectioned

1 ripe medium banana, peeled and sliced

1 cup blueberries

½ cup unsweetened, unflavored rice milk

½ cup cooked rice

Nut-free
Vegan

REPAIR

Breakfast

PER SERVING
CALORIES: 503
CARBS: 119G
FAT: 2G
PROTEIN: 8G
SUGAR: 51G

1. In a blender, combine the orange, banana, blueberries, rice milk, and rice.

2. Blend the mixture until it is smooth and frothy.

3. Serve immediately.

Green Tea Smoothie

SERVES 1 / PREP TIME: 5 MINUTES

Green tea is high in natural antioxidants. Regular green tea does contain caffeine, so on this diet, make sure you buy decaffeinated green tea. You can also substitute any variety of decaffeinated tea for the green tea.

Ingredient tip: *To keep the delicate flavor of the smoothie, look for white or oolong tea, or select a spicy herbal tea such as cinnamon. Unsweetened frozen peaches make a good substitute for fresh peaches.*

1 cup brewed decaffeinated green tea, chilled

1 peach, pitted and cut into chunks

½ banana

½ cup cooked brown rice

1. In a blender, combine the tea, peach, banana, and rice.

2. Blend until smooth.

3. Serve immediately.

Nut-free
Vegan

REPAIR

Breakfast

PER SERVING
CALORIES: 263
CARBS: 59G
FAT: 2G
PROTEIN: 5G
SUGAR: 15G

Spiced Baked Apples with Flax

SERVES 4 / PREP TIME: 5 MINUTES / COOK TIME: 35 MINUTES

Flax is one of the oldest fiber crops in the world. It plays a part in many old-fashioned fairy tales. Today, flax is treasured for its seeds, which contain high amounts of healthy omega-3 fatty acids.

Ingredient tip: *Choose a sweet-tart baking apple such as Pink Lady, Braeburn, Granny Smith, or Honey crisp. All of these apples hold up well to baking and have delicious flavor.*

4 apples, cored but not peeled

1 teaspoon ground cinnamon, divided

½ teaspoon ground nutmeg, divided

½ teaspoon ground mace, divided

4 tablespoons ground golden flaxseed, divided

Nut-free
Paleo-friendly
Vegan

REPAIR

Breakfast

PER SERVING
CALORIES: 136
CARBS: 28G
FAT: 2G
PROTEIN: 1G
SUGAR: 19G

1. Preheat the oven to 400°F.
2. Put the apples in a 9-by-13-inch baking dish, and stuff each with ¼ teaspoon cinnamon, ⅛ teaspoon nutmeg, and ⅛ teaspoon mace.
3. Add enough water to the baking dish to cover the bottom of the pan.
4. Cover the dish with foil, and bake the apples until they are tender, 25 to 35 minutes.
5. Remove the apples from the oven, and top each with 1 tablespoon flaxseed.

Apple and Pear "Pie"

SERVES 2 / PREP TIME: 10 MINUTES, PLUS 1 TO 2 HOURS CHILLING TIME /
COOK TIME: 20 MINUTES

*Slicing apples and pears and pressing them into a round pie plate or a tart pan
gives this dish a classic "pie" appearance. If you don't have a pie plate, press the
fruit into a round cake pan or even a rimmed dinner plate.*

Serving tip: *Serve slices of this "pie" alongside scrambled egg whites, which will
provide you with plenty of lean protein to make it through the morning.*

2 apples, peeled, cored, and cut into ½-inch chunks

1 pear, peeled, cored, and cut into ½-inch chunks

1 tablespoon grated fresh ginger

½ teaspoon ground cinnamon

¼ teaspoon ground nutmeg

Pinch ground cloves

Unsweetened, unflavored rice milk, for serving

Nut-free
Vegan

REPAIR

Breakfast

PER SERVING
CALORIES: 208
CARBS: 51G
FAT: 1G
PROTEIN: 1G
SUGAR: 31G

1. Fill a medium stockpot with water, and place it over medium-high heat.
   When the water is hot but not boiling, add the apples, cover the pot, and
   cook until they are nearly tender, about 10 minutes.

2. Reduce the heat to medium-low. Add the pears to the pot. Cover and cook
   for 5 minutes.

3. When the apples and pears are tender, use a slotted spoon to transfer
   them to a large bowl. Mash them well with a fork.

4. Stir in the ginger, cinnamon, nutmeg, and cloves. Stir well to combine;
   then gently press the fruit into a pie plate. Cover and chill in the
   refrigerator for 1 to 2 hours.

5. Slice and serve topped with unsweetened rice milk.

Coconut Yogurt and Melon Parfait

SERVES 1 / PREP TIME: 10 MINUTES

Many grocery stores offer yogurt made from coconut in the dairy section. Choose unsweetened, plain coconut yogurt for these parfaits. Flavored and fruit-on-the-bottom yogurts contain added sugar. If you can't find coconut yogurt, try almond yogurt. If your local grocer doesn't carry it, your local health food store or co-op most likely will.

Substitution tip: *Use any seasonal fresh, juicy fruit in these parfaits in place of the melon. Consider plums, peaches, nectarines, berries, or pluots as a delicious and nutritious substitution.*

1 (6-ounce) container plain coconut yogurt
½ teaspoon ground cinnamon
1 packet stevia
½ cup honeydew, cut into ½-inch cubes
½ cup cantaloupe, cut into ½-inch cubes

1. In a small bowl, combine the yogurt, cinnamon, and stevia. Whisk to incorporate the ingredients.

2. In a parfait glass or dessert dish, layer the yogurt mixture, honeydew, and cantaloupe in three or four alternating layers.

3. Serve cold.

Nut-free
Paleo-friendly
Vegan

REPAIR

Breakfast

PER SERVING
CALORIES: 135
CARBS: 26G
FAT: 6G
PROTEIN: 1G
SUGAR: 15G

Breakfast Rice

SERVES 4 / PREP TIME: 5 MINUTES / COOK TIME: 10 MINUTES

Kale is a nutritional powerhouse that is available year-round at every supermarket in the country. Look for packaged kale or baby kale in the refrigerated section of the produce aisle. Wash the kale thoroughly to remove any dirt and grit.

¼ cup low-sodium vegetable broth

3½ cups cooked brown rice

2 scallions, sliced

1 tablespoon rice wine vinegar

1 tablespoon gluten-free soy sauce

1 (5-ounce) bag chopped fresh kale leaves

2 egg whites

Fine sea salt

Freshly ground black pepper

Nut-free
Vegetarian

REPAIR

Breakfast

PER SERVING
CALORIES: 637
CARBS: 131G
FAT: 5G
PROTEIN: 16G
SUGAR: 0G

1. In a large nonstick skillet, heat the broth over medium-high heat.

2. Stir in the rice, scallions, vinegar, and soy sauce. Cook until the rice is heated through, about 3 minutes.

3. Add the kale and cook until it wilts, 2 to 3 minutes longer.

4. Push the cooked rice mixture to the sides of the skillet. Add the egg whites to the center of the skillet. Cook the eggs, stirring frequently, until set, about 2 minutes.

5. Mix the eggs with the rice. Season the mixture with salt and pepper.

Slow Cooker Cranberry-Orange Oatmeal

SERVES 4 / PREP TIME: 5 MINUTES / COOK TIME: 8 HOURS IN A SLOW COOKER

Put this delicious and nourishing oatmeal in your slow cooker just before you go to bed, and you'll wake up to a hot, healthy breakfast that's sure to get your day started just right. This recipe uses steel-cut oats, and it has warm spices and delicious fruit flavors that will wake up your palate. Plus, it has beneficial fiber and slow-burning carbohydrates that will keep your energy high throughout the morning.

Ingredient tip: *Many brands of oatmeal are processed in plants that also process gluten grains, or the oats grow in fields next to wheat or barley crops, so they are cross-contaminated with gluten. Make sure you buy gluten-free oats for this recipe.*

1 cup gluten-free steel-cut oats

3 cups orange juice

1 cup water

2 packets stevia

¼ teaspoon fresh grated nutmeg

½ teaspoon ground cinnamon

Pinch of salt

1 cup fresh cranberries

1. In the slow cooker, mix together the oats, orange juice, water, stevia, nutmeg, cinnamon, salt, and cranberries.

2. Cover and cook on low for 8 hours.

Nut-free
Vegan

REPAIR

Breakfast

PER SERVING
CALORIES: 174
CARBS: 37G
FAT: 2G
PROTEIN: 4G
SUGAR: 17G

Hot Quinoa Breakfast Cereal with Flax

SERVES 4 / PREP TIME: 5 MINUTES / COOK TIME: 25 MINUTES

Look for quinoa in the bulk section of natural foods stores. You can also find it in the grain or gluten-free section of your favorite market. Spread any extra cooked quinoa on a baking sheet to cool. It will retain its texture and taste even better as leftovers.

Time-saving tip: *Flaked quinoa, which contains the endosperm and the bran, is considered a whole grain. It provides the same nutritional benefits as whole-grain quinoa, and cooks in just under 1 minute in boiling water. If you are using flaked quinoa, boil the water, add it to the quinoa in a heat-proof bowl, stir, and allow it to rest for 1 minute before proceeding with step 2.*

Nut-free
Vegan

REPAIR

Breakfast

PER SERVING
CALORIES: 392
CARBS: 66G
FAT: 8G
PROTEIN: 13G
SUGAR: 6G

2 cups water

1 cup quinoa

Pinch fine sea salt

½ teaspoon ground cinnamon

⅛ teaspoon ground nutmeg

2 tablespoons flaxseed

1 cup unsweetened, unflavored rice milk

1. In a medium saucepan, bring the water to a rolling boil over medium-high heat.

2. Add the quinoa and salt. Return to a boil; then simmer gently until the water is completely absorbed, about 20 minutes. Remove from the heat and allow to rest for 5 minutes.

3. Stir in the cinnamon, nutmeg, flaxseed, and rice milk.

Almond Butter and Banana Toast

SERVES 1 / PREP TIME: 2 MINUTES

Almond butter makes a delicious substitute for peanut butter. Almonds are high in beneficial omega-3 fatty acids and also contain vitamin E, magnesium, riboflavin, and manganese. Choose any gluten-free sandwich bread, which you can find in the bread or freezer section at your local grocery store.

Technique tip: *It's easy to make your own almond butter, if you wish. Simply put 1 cup of almonds in a food processor and process until you have a smooth butter, stopping occasionally to scrape down the sides. The process will take 15 to 20 minutes. If you'd like to make it a little bit chunky, stir in chopped almonds. Almond butter will keep in the refrigerator for up to one week.*

1 slice gluten-free sandwich bread

1 tablespoon unsweetened, unsalted almond butter

½ banana, sliced

1. Toast the sandwich bread to the desired level of darkness.

2. Spread the almond butter on top of the warm toast.

3. Top with the banana slices.

Vegan

REPAIR

Breakfast

PER SERVING
CALORIES: 304
CARBS: 40G
FAT: 14G
PROTEIN: 7G
SUGAR: 10G

Pumpkin Pancakes

SERVES 4 / PREP TIME: 10 MINUTES / COOK TIME: 10 MINUTES

Just because you can't eat wheat for four weeks doesn't mean you must give up pancakes. These wheat-free pancakes use baked potato and gluten-free flour in place of wheat flour. The result is a light and tender pancake. To keep the pancakes tender, do not overmix the ingredients in step 3. The final batter will have streaks and lumps in it. Overmixing will yield a tough, rubbery pancake.

Substitution tip: *While this recipe calls for gluten-free all-purpose flour, any wheat-free flour will do. If you have rice flour, potato flour, or some other wheat-free flour, you can replace it in this recipe at a one-to-one ratio.*

Nut-free
Vegetarian

REPAIR

Breakfast

PER SERVING
CALORIES: 328
CARBS: 67G
FAT: 2G
PROTEIN: 11G
SUGAR: 5G

½ cup baked russet potato flesh (or any starchy potato), cooled

1 cup gluten-free all-purpose flour

½ cup quick-cooking oats

2 teaspoons baking powder

½ teaspoon ground cinnamon

⅛ teaspoon ground nutmeg

⅛ teaspoon ground ginger

⅛ teaspoon ground allspice

7 egg whites

1 cup canned unsweetened pumpkin purée

¾ cup unsweetened, unflavored rice milk

1 teaspoon vanilla extract

1. In a large bowl, whisk together the baked potato, flour, oats, baking powder, cinnamon, nutmeg, ginger, and allspice until well combined.

2. In a separate bowl, whisk together the egg whites, pumpkin, rice milk, and vanilla.

3. Use a rubber spatula to create a well in the center of the dry ingredients. Pour the wet ingredients into the well and then carefully fold the mixture until it is just combined. Some streaks of flour will remain. Do not overmix.

4. Heat a nonstick sauté pan or griddle over medium-high heat.

5. Scoop or pour the batter into the heated pan, using about ¼ cup for each pancake.

6. Cook each pancake on one side until bubbles begin to form in the wet batter on top. Flip the pancake and cook for about 3 more minutes, until it springs back to the touch.

Dutch Apple Pancake

SERVES 4 / PREP TIME: 15 MINUTES / COOK TIME: 15 MINUTES

In this recipe, gluten-free batter puffs appealingly around sweet-tart apples. With the sweetness of the apples, the pancake requires no additional toppings. Select a sweet-tart apple, like a Pink Lady, Braeburn, Gala, or Honeycrisp. You can use any gluten-free all-purpose flour, which you can find in many grocery and health food stores.

⅔ cup gluten-free all-purpose flour

½ teaspoon baking powder

1 teaspoon ground cinnamon, divided

Pinch salt

4 eggs

4 tablespoons unsweetened, unflavored almond or coconut milk

6 tablespoons extra-virgin coconut oil, melted and slightly cooled, divided

1 teaspoon vanilla extract

½ teaspoon fresh grated nutmeg

1 large apple, peeled, cored, and sliced

Nut-free

Vegetarian

REPAIR

Breakfast

PER SERVING

CALORIES: 392

CARBS: 23G

FAT: 29G

PROTEIN: 8G

SUGAR: 5G

1. Preheat the oven to 450°F.

2. In a blender, combine the flour, baking powder, ½ teaspoon cinnamon, salt, eggs, almond milk, 2 tablespoons coconut oil, and vanilla. Blend the ingredients until a thin, smooth batter forms. Set aside.

3. Meanwhile, heat the remaining 4 tablespoons coconut oil in a 10-inch ovenproof sauté pan over medium-high heat.

4. Sprinkle the remaining ½ teaspoon cinnamon and the nutmeg over the melted coconut oil, and add the apples in a circular pattern along the bottom of the pan.

5. Cook without stirring the apples for 3 minutes. Turn off the heat.

6. Carefully pour the batter over the top of the apples.

7. Transfer the pan to the oven. Bake until the batter puffs and is golden, about 15 minutes. Cut into wedges and serve.

French Toast with Warm Berry Compote

SERVES 4 / PREP TIME: 15 MINUTES / COOK TIME: 10 MINUTES

Top this tasty French toast with a spicy warm berry compote for a delicious and satisfying start to your day. Use any gluten-free sandwich bread for this recipe. When making French toast, many people just give the bread a quick dip in the custard before cooking it, but that doesn't allow the bread to completely soak up the custard. Instead, soak it for three or four minutes per side to allow it to completely absorb the tasty custard.

2 eggs plus 2 egg whites, beaten
1 cup unsweetened coconut milk
1 teaspoon vanilla extract
Zest of 1 orange
½ teaspoon fresh grated nutmeg, divided
4 slices gluten-free sandwich bread
2 cups blackberries, frozen or fresh
2 cups blueberries, frozen or fresh
½ teaspoon ground cinnamon
Pinch of salt
1 teaspoon arrowroot powder
Juice of 1 orange
1 tablespoon coconut oil

**Nut-free
Vegetarian**

REPAIR

Breakfast

PER SERVING
CALORIES: 429
CARBS: 48G
FAT: 24G
PROTEIN: 10G
SUGAR: 18G

1. In a medium bowl, combine the beaten eggs, coconut milk, vanilla, orange zest, and ¼ teaspoon nutmeg. Whisk until well combined. Pour the mixture into a shallow dish.

2. Put the slices of bread in the dish, and allow them to soak up the custard, about 3 minutes per side.

3. While the bread soaks, combine the blackberries, blueberries, cinnamon, salt, and remaining ¼ teaspoon nutmeg in a medium pot.

4. Heat the pot over medium-high heat, stirring frequently, until it comes to a boil. Reduce the heat to a simmer, stirring frequently, to allow the juices of the berries to release, about 5 minutes. »

French Toast with Warm Berry Compote *continued*

5. In a small bowl, whisk together the arrowroot powder and orange juice. Stirring constantly, carefully pour the slurry into the berry mixture. Simmer until the berry sauce thickens.

6. In a large sauté pan or skillet, melt the coconut oil over medium-high heat, spreading it to coat the pan.

7. Cook the soaked bread until it is golden on both sides, about 4 minutes per side.

8. Serve the French toast topped with the berry compote.

Sweet Potato Waffles

SERVES 4 / PREP TIME: 10 MINUTES / COOK TIME: 20 MINUTES

Grated sweet potatoes replace flour in these simple waffles. Any type of fresh sweet potatoes or yams will do. You can also replace the sweet potatoes with butternut squash or pumpkin. If you don't like nuts, omit the pecans. Or you can substitute walnuts for the pecans. To make the waffles Paleo-friendly, brush the waffle iron with extra-virgin coconut oil or pastured butter. Otherwise, use any oil you wish to prepare the waffle iron.

Technique tip: *If you don't have a waffle iron, drop the mixture into a greased, warm nonstick pan and cook as you would a pancake, over medium-high heat for about 4 minutes per side.*

**Paleo-friendly
Vegetarian**

REPAIR

Breakfast

PER SERVING
CALORIES: 173
CARBS: 23G
FAT: 5G
PROTEIN: 10G
SUGAR: 1G

4 eggs

4 egg whites

2 teaspoons ground cinnamon

½ teaspoon ground nutmeg

½ teaspoon ground ginger

½ teaspoon ground cloves

Pinch of salt

2 large raw sweet potatoes, peeled and finely grated

½ cup finely chopped pecans

Oil or butter, for brushing

1. In a medium bowl, whisk together the eggs, egg whites, cinnamon, nutmeg, ginger, cloves, and salt.

2. Stir in the sweet potatoes and pecans. Mix well.

3. Heat the waffle iron on high. When the waffle iron is heated, brush it liberally with oil.

4. Pour the batter by half cupfuls onto the prepared waffle iron. Cook until the batter sets, about 5 minutes.

Minted Cantaloupe and Cucumber Salad

SERVES 4 / PREP TIME: 15 MINUTES

This salad is ideal for the summer and early fall, when cantaloupe and cucumber are at their peak of ripeness. You can use tart apples, such as Granny Smith, in place of the jicama for a different flavor profile. Choose fresh young corn, which is surprisingly good uncooked.

1 medium jicama, cut into ½-inch dice

1 cup 1-inch cantaloupe chunks

½ cucumber, peeled and cut into ½-inch dice

Kernels from 2 ears of corn

Zest and fruit of 1 navel orange

Zest and juice of 1 lime

10 fresh mint leaves, cut into slivers

¼ teaspoon ground cinnamon

¼ teaspoon fine sea salt

Nut-free
Paleo-friendly
Vegan

REPAIR

Lunch

PER SERVING
CALORIES: 145
CARBS: 34G
FAT: 1G
PROTEIN: 4G
SUGAR: 12G

1. In a medium bowl, combine the jicama, cantaloupe, cucumber, and corn.

2. Zest the orange into the mixture. Then cut off the orange peel and slice the flesh into ½-inch rounds.

3. Stir the orange rounds, lime zest and juice, mint, cinnamon, and salt into the fruit and vegetable mixture.

4. Toss gently before serving.

Tomato and Orange Chopped Salad

SERVES 2 / PREP TIME: 10 MINUTES

You can add any vegetable to a chopped salad. Romaine hearts, green beans, and snap peas would all make fine additions. Zest the orange for the dressing; then peel and section the orange for the salad.

1 navel orange

Juice of 2 limes

¼ teaspoon kosher salt

⅛ teaspoon freshly ground black pepper

⅛ teaspoon ground cinnamon

⅛ teaspoon ground cumin

1 yellow bell pepper, seeded and diced

1 large beefsteak tomato, seeded and cut into ¼-inch dice

½ cucumber, diced

¼ cup finely diced red onion

1 (14-ounce) can hearts of palm, drained and sliced

1. Zest the orange into a small bowl. Whisk in the lime juice, salt, pepper, cinnamon, and cumin. Set the dressing aside.

2. Peel the orange and divide the flesh into sections. In a large bowl, combine the orange sections, bell pepper, tomato, cucumber, onion, and hearts of palm.

3. Pour the dressing over the salad and toss to combine.

Nut-free
Paleo-friendly
Vegan

REPAIR

Lunch

PER SERVING
CALORIES: 151
CARBS: 31G
FAT: 2G
PROTEIN: 8G
SUGAR: 14G

Gingered Peach and Rice Salad

SERVES 4 / PREP TIME: 5 MINUTES

Cook the rice and prepare the fruit the night before, and this dish comes together very quickly. You can use any fruits or vegetables that are in season and appeal to you. For instance, in autumn and winter, substitute apples and pears for the peaches and grapes.

Nut-free
Vegan

REPAIR

Lunch

PER SERVING
CALORIES: 230
CARBS: 53G
FAT: 1G
PROTEIN: 4G
SUGAR: 14G

Zest of 1 lime
1 tablespoon honey
1 tablespoon low-sodium vegetable broth
½ teaspoon ground ginger
Pinch ground cinnamon
2 cups cooked long-grain rice
3 peaches or nectarines, pitted and cut into bite-size pieces
1 cup seedless grapes, halved

1. In a medium bowl, whisk together the lime zest, honey, broth, ginger, and cinnamon.
2. Add the rice and fruit, and stir to combine.

Quinoa Salad with Lemon and Peppers

SERVES 6 / PREP TIME: 20 MINUTES

To make this salad, cook your quinoa ahead of time and chill it in the refrigerator for several hours or overnight. Quinoa can have a bitter taste, but rinsing the dry quinoa well before cooking washes away most of the bitter residue. Place the uncooked quinoa in a fine mesh sieve, and run it under cold water for a few minutes to remove all of the bitter residue.

Technique tip: Cook large batches of quinoa, and freeze individual portions in tightly sealed containers for up to six months. Then all you need to do is thaw some quinoa to make a healthy salad. To cook quinoa, put one part quinoa to two parts water in a large pot and simmer, uncovered, over medium-low heat, stirring occasionally, until it is tender, about 15 to 20 minutes.

2 cups cooked quinoa, chilled

1 red bell pepper, seeded and chopped

4 scallions, chopped

12 cherry tomatoes, halved

1 (14-ounce) can artichoke hearts, drained

¼ cup freshly squeezed lemon juice

½ cup extra-virgin olive oil

3 garlic cloves, finely minced

½ teaspoon Dijon mustard

½ teaspoon sea salt

¼ teaspoon freshly ground black pepper

1. In a large bowl, combine the quinoa, bell pepper, scallions, tomatoes, and artichoke hearts.

2. In a small bowl, whisk together the lemon juice, olive oil, garlic, mustard, salt, and pepper until it emulsifies.

3. Pour the vinaigrette over the quinoa, and toss to combine. Serve immediately.

**Nut-free
Vegan**

REPAIR

Lunch

PER SERVING
CALORIES: 408
CARBS: 49G
FAT: 21G
PROTEIN: 11G
SUGAR: 8G

Pesto Chicken Pasta Salad

SERVES 6 / PREP TIME: 20 MINUTES / COOK TIME: 15 MINUTES

Cook the pasta ahead of time, and chill it for this pasta salad. If you like, you can make a large batch of pasta and freeze any leftovers for future use. Select any gluten-free rotini pasta. You can find gluten-free rotini in the pasta aisle of many grocery stores or at your local health food store.

Time-saving tip: *Use cooked deli counter chicken for this salad to save time. This recipe also works well with leftover chicken or turkey.*

2 cups gluten-free rotini pasta

½ red onion, very thinly sliced

3 plum tomatoes, chopped

½ cup sliced black pitted olives, drained

2 cups cooked skinless chicken breast, cut into cubes

2 cups baby spinach leaves

½ cup fresh basil

½ cup walnuts

3 garlic cloves

2 tablespoons red wine vinegar

2 tablespoons extra-virgin olive oil

½ teaspoon fine sea salt

¼ teaspoon freshly ground black pepper

PER SERVING
CALORIES: 297
CARBS: 20G
FAT: 16G
PROTEIN: 20G
SUGAR: 3G

1. Fill a large pot with water and heat it over high heat until it boils. Stir in the pasta and return to a boil. Boil the pasta according to the package directions, until al dente.

2. Drain the pasta in a colander, and put it in the refrigerator in a sealed container to chill.

3. In a large bowl, combine the chilled cooked pasta, red onion, tomatoes, olives, and chicken, stirring to mix.

4. In the bowl of a food processor or a blender, combine the spinach, basil, walnuts, garlic, red wine vinegar, olive oil, salt, and pepper. Process until it forms a smooth, slightly watery paste, about one minute.

5. Pour the pesto over the pasta, and toss to combine.

Gazpacho

SERVES 4 / PREP TIME: 10 MINUTES

This cold soup has its roots in southern Spain, where the summers are dry and hot. You can add almost any vegetable to this dish to make it your own. You can also make this soup in Stage Two of your diet by adding poached shrimp. In Stage Three, add shrimp and diced avocado or slivered, toasted almonds.

Substitution tip: *Replace the fire-roasted tomatoes with three large heirloom tomatoes. In-season heirloom tomatoes have a sweetness and richness that just can't be captured in canned tomatoes, so the result will be a very fresh-tasting gazpacho.*

2 (15-ounce) cans fire-roasted whole tomatoes, with juice

1 cucumber, peeled, seeded, and chopped, divided

1 garlic clove, minced

2 scallions, coarsely chopped

3 tablespoons red wine vinegar

½ teaspoon fine sea salt

¼ teaspoon freshly ground black pepper

Dash cayenne pepper

¼ cup fresh basil leaves, cut into thin ribbons

1. In the bowl of a food processor or a blender, process the tomatoes and their juice, half the chopped cucumber, the garlic, scallions, red wine vinegar, salt, pepper, and cayenne. Pulse until vegetables just begin to come together, about 1 minute. Do not purée.

2. Divide the soup among 4 serving bowls.

3. Garnish each with some basil ribbons and the remaining half of the chopped cucumber.

Nut-free
Paleo-friendly
Vegan

REPAIR

Lunch

PER SERVING
CALORIES: 56
CARBS: 12G
FAT: 1G
PROTEIN: 3G
SUGAR: 6G

Easy Chicken Rice Soup

SERVES 4 / PREP TIME: 10 MINUTES / COOK TIME: 15 MINUTES

This chicken and rice soup comes together quickly and is very flavorful. Instead of celery, fennel root adds an interesting anise-like flavor to this soup. If you'd like a spicier soup, add hot sauce just before serving.

2 tablespoons olive oil

8 ounces boneless, skinless chicken breast, cut into ½-inch pieces

1 onion, chopped

1 carrot, peeled and chopped

½ fennel bulb, chopped

12 shiitake mushrooms, stemmed and sliced

3 garlic cloves, minced

6 cups low-sodium chicken broth

1 cup cooked brown rice

Fine sea salt

Freshly ground black pepper

Nut-free

REPAIR

Lunch

PER SERVING
CALORIES: 409
CARBS: 56G
FAT: 10G
PROTEIN: 27G
SUGAR: 10G

1. In a large stockpot, heat the olive oil over medium-high heat until it shimmers. Add the chicken and cook, stirring frequently, until it is browned and cooked through, about 6 minutes.

2. Remove the chicken from the oil with tongs, and set it aside on a platter.

3. Add the onion, carrot, fennel, and mushrooms to the oil remaining in the pot. Cook, stirring frequently, until the vegetables soften and begin to brown, about 6 minutes.

4. Add the garlic and cook, stirring constantly, until it is fragrant, about 30 seconds.

5. Add the broth, and use a spoon to scrape any browned bits off the bottom of the pan.

6. Add the rice and reserved chicken. Cook until the rice and chicken heat through, about 2 more minutes. Season with salt and pepper.

Thai Rice Noodle Soup with Turkey

SERVES 4 / PREP TIME: 15 MINUTES / COOK TIME: 20 MINUTES

This warming soup uses pad Thai rice noodles, which you can find in the Asian section of your grocery store. Read the label to make sure you purchase noodles made only with rice flour and no added wheat. The flavor profile of the soup also relies heavily on ginger and garlic, a delicious Asian combination.

Ingredient tip: *Thai rice noodles generally don't require any cooking. Instead, you just soak them in hot liquid (water or broth) for 5 to 8 minutes, and they soften. Although this recipe has general instructions for the rice noodles, follow those on the package.*

2 tablespoons coconut oil

1 teaspoon sesame oil

6 scallions, chopped

1 tablespoon grated fresh ginger

2 carrots, peeled and sliced

3 garlic cloves, minced

4 cups low-sodium chicken broth

1 tablespoon rice vinegar

1 cup bok choy, chopped

2 cups cooked turkey, cubed

8 ounces pad Thai rice noodles

Sea salt

Freshly ground black pepper

Nut-free

REPAIR

Lunch

PER SERVING
CALORIES: 467
CARBS: 57G
FAT: 13G
PROTEIN: 28G
SUGAR: 3G

1. In a large pot, heat the coconut and sesame oils over medium-high heat until they shimmer.

2. Add the scallions, ginger, and carrots, and cook, stirring occasionally, until the vegetables are soft and beginning to brown, 5 to 7 minutes.

3. Stir in the garlic and cook, stirring constantly, until the garlic is fragrant, about 30 seconds. »

4. Add the broth, rice vinegar, bok choy, and turkey, and bring the soup to a boil. Reduce the heat to medium, and simmer for 5 minutes, stirring occasionally, to allow the flavors to blend and the bok choy to soften.

5. Take the pot off the heat, and stir in the rice noodles. Cover and soak until the noodles soften, about 5 to 8 minutes (check noodle package for specific times).

6. Season with salt and pepper.

REPAIR

Lunch

Open-Faced Prosciutto, Fig, and Arugula Sandwich

SERVES 4 / PREP TIME: 15 MINUTES / COOK TIME: 6 MINUTES

Use hearty gluten-free sandwich bread for these sandwiches. Many people think Ezekiel bread is gluten- and wheat-free, but it's not. It contains spelt, which is actually hulled wheat. You can find truly wheat-free, gluten-free bread at the local health food store, but it may also be available in the freezer section of your grocery store.

Substitution tip: *If you can't find fresh figs, you can use sliced pears or another seasonal fruit. To substitute for prosciutto, choose thin slices of turkey ham.*

4 slices gluten-free sandwich bread

2 tablespoons extra-virgin olive oil

4 thin slices prosciutto

8 fresh figs, quartered

Zest of 1 lemon

2 tablespoons honey

1 tablespoon minced shallot

1 tablespoon minced fresh thyme

Fine sea salt

Freshly ground black pepper

4 ounces baby arugula

Nut-free

REPAIR

Lunch

PER SERVING
CALORIES: 338
CARBS: 48G
FAT: 14G
PROTEIN: 11G
SUGAR: 32G

1. Preheat the broiler. Brush both sides of the bread with olive oil, and place it under the broiler until it browns on both sides, about 3 minutes per side.

2. Place a slice of prosciutto on each piece of toast.

3. In a medium bowl, combine the figs, lemon zest, honey, shallot, and thyme, and stir. Season with salt and pepper.

4. Divide the mixture evenly among the 4 sandwiches. Top with the arugula.

Chicken and Grape Salad Sandwich

SERVES 1 / PREP TIME: 15 MINUTES

Eliminate the sugar and high-fructose corn syrup found in commercial processed mayonnaise by making your own Easy Homemade Mayonnaise (page 37). Mix this creamy and delicious mayonnaise with savory chicken and sweet grapes, along with crunchy celery, for a satisfying and healthy sandwich.

¼ cup cooked skinless chicken, chilled and cut into ½-inch cubes
½ celery stalk, minced
10 seedless grapes, halved
1 scallion, minced
2 tablespoons Easy Homemade Mayonnaise
Pinch of salt
Freshly ground black pepper
1 slice gluten-free sandwich bread, toasted

Nut-free

REPAIR

Lunch

PER SERVING
CALORIES: 270
CARBS: 25G
FAT: 13G
PROTEIN: 13G
SUGAR: 7G

1. In a small bowl, combine the chicken, celery, grapes, scallion, mayonnaise, salt, and pepper until well mixed.

2. Cut the bread in half and top one half with the chicken salad. Cover with the other half slice of bread.

Chicken Breasts with Blackberry Sauce

SERVES 2 / PREP TIME: 10 MINUTES / COOK TIME: 25 MINUTES

You can use fresh or thawed frozen blackberries for this delicious baked chicken. Use two boneless, skinless chicken breast halves or one whole boneless, skinless chicken breast, cut in half. The addition of spices to the blackberries imparts savoriness to the sweetness of the blackberries, which perfectly complements the chicken.

2 (5-ounce) boneless, skinless chicken breast halves
Sea salt
Freshly ground black pepper
¼ cup blackberries
¼ cup low-sodium chicken broth
2 garlic cloves, finely minced
1 tablespoon minced shallot
¼ teaspoon dried thyme
1 tablespoon red wine vinegar
Dash red pepper flakes

1. Preheat the oven to 375°F.

2. Season the chicken breasts with sea salt and black pepper. Place them in a 9-by-9-inch baking dish, and bake until the juices run clear, about 20 to 25 minutes.

3. Meanwhile, in a medium saucepan, heat the blackberries, broth, garlic, shallot, thyme, vinegar, and red pepper flakes over medium-high heat until the mixture simmers. Reduce the heat to medium-low.

4. Cook, stirring frequently and mashing the blackberries with the spoon, until the liquid reduces by half, about 10 minutes.

5. Serve the chicken sliced with the blackberry sauce spooned over the top.

Nut-free

REPAIR

Lunch

PER SERVING
CALORIES: 292
CARBS: 4G
FAT: 11G
PROTEIN: 42G
SUGAR: 1G

Pork Tenderloin with Mustard and Plums

SERVES 4 / PREP TIME: 15 MINUTES / COOK TIME: 25 MINUTES

Pork and mustard are a delicious combination, and the plums add sweetness to this recipe. Read the ingredients on the mustard jar carefully to make sure you don't buy a brand that contains wheat or sugar.

Nonstick cooking spray

1¼ pounds pork tenderloin

Fine sea salt

Freshly ground black pepper

1 tablespoon coarse grain mustard

1 tablespoon Dijon mustard

4 plums, pitted and coarsely chopped

1 navel orange, zested, peeled, and segmented

1 onion, chopped

Nut-free
Paleo-friendly

REPAIR

Lunch

PER SERVING
CALORIES: 262
CARBS: 13G
FAT: 6G
PROTEIN: 38G
SUGAR: 10G

1. Preheat the oven to 375°F.

2. Spray an oven-safe skillet with cooking spray, and heat it over medium-high heat.

3. Season the pork with salt and pepper. Add the pork to the skillet and cook, without turning, until it begins to caramelize, about 4 minutes per side. Remove the pan from the heat.

4. Spread both mustards on top of the pork. Scatter the plums, orange zest, orange sections, and onion in the pan around the pork.

5. Roast until the pork's internal temperature reaches 140°F, 15 to 18 minutes.

6. Remove the pan from the oven, and allow the pork to rest for 10 minutes before carving. Serve the meat topped with the roasted plums and oranges.

Herbal Tea Smoothie

SERVES 4 / PREP TIME: 5 MINUTES

To give this smoothie a thicker consistency, add a banana to the blender. The recipe also works with decaffeinated black tea or red rooibos tea. In summer, make this smoothie with fresh peaches and sun tea. You can also use frozen mango for a more tropical flavor.

Ingredient tip: *Different brands and forms of stevia have different levels of sweetness. Choose a brand you like, and then determine the right amount of sweetness that works for you. Start by adding a little stevia and tasting, and then add more as needed.*

2 cups frozen unsweetened peaches

¾ cup chamomile tea, chilled

Juice of 1 lemon

¼ teaspoon powdered stevia

1. In a blender, combine the peaches, tea, lemon juice, and stevia.
2. Blend until smooth and frothy. Serve immediately.

Nut-free
Paleo-friendly
Vegan

REPAIR

Snacks

PER SERVING
CALORIES: 31
CARBS: 5G
FAT: 0G
PROTEIN: 1G
SUGAR: 4G

Piña Colada Chia Smoothie

SERVES 2 / PREP TIME: 10 MINUTES

Have a taste of the tropics with this delicious fruit smoothie that makes a great afternoon pick-me-up. With the tasty flavors of piña colada—pineapple and coconut—this creamy smoothie gives you a small tropical vacation in the middle of the day. Plus, it's loaded with vitamins and it tastes great.

Substitution tip: *Feel free to substitute almond milk for coconut milk. Likewise, mix and match different tropical fruits, such as mango or papaya.*

2 tablespoons chia seeds

1 cup unsweetened coconut milk

1 cup frozen unsweetened pineapple chunks

1 teaspoon rum flavoring (optional)

Nut-free
Vegan

REPAIR

Snacks

PER SERVING
CALORIES: 271
CARBS: 26G
FAT: 15G
PROTEIN: 8G
SUGAR: 8G

1. In a small measuring cup, combine the chia seeds and coconut milk. Allow the seeds to soak in the coconut milk for 20 minutes, until they become gelatinous.

2. Pour the mixture into a blender. Add the pineapple chunks and rum flavoring, if using.

3. Blend until smooth.

Chocolate Shake

SERVES 1 / PREP TIME: 5 MINUTES

This quick shake is just as delicious as a chocolate milkshake, but doesn't contain dairy or refined sugar. Use 1 tablespoon pure maple syrup to sweeten it if you don't enjoy the taste of stevia. Be sure to use pure maple syrup and not maple-flavored syrup, which contains refined sugar.

1 banana, peeled and frozen

1 cup plain, unsweetened coconut yogurt

½ cup unsweetened, unflavored rice milk

3 tablespoons unsweetened cocoa powder

½ teaspoon powdered stevia

1. In a blender, combine the banana, coconut yogurt, rice milk, cocoa powder, and stevia.

2. Blend until smooth.

Nut-free
Vegan

REPAIR

Snacks

PER SERVING
CALORIES: 302
CARBS: 60G
FAT: 11G
PROTEIN: 5G
SUGAR: 22G

Carrot and Fruit Salad

SERVES 4 / PREP TIME: 15 MINUTES

Carrots have a sweet, starchy taste that goes well with fruit. This sweet salad also has healthy apples, sweet fennel, and soft Asian pears for a delicious blend that offers a variety of textures, from juicy and soft to crunchy. To make the salad colorful, look for brightly colored heirloom carrots in red, purple, and white at your local farmers' market. For the best flavor, serve this salad chilled.

Ingredient tip: *Using both the fennel bulb and the fronds adds a lovely anise flavor to this juicy fruit salad.*

Nut-free
Paleo-friendly
Vegan

REPAIR

Snacks

PER SERVING
CALORIES: 122
CARBS: 30G
FAT: 0G
PROTEIN: 2G
SUGAR: 15G

4 carrots, peeled and grated

½ bulb fennel, thinly sliced

1 apple, cored and thinly sliced

1 Asian pear, cored and thinly sliced

½ jicama, peeled and julienned

2 tablespoons chopped fresh fennel fronds

Juice of 1 lime

1. In a medium bowl, combine the carrots, fennel bulb, apple, pear, jicama, and fennel fronds. Stir well to combine.

2. Squeeze the lime over the top of the salad, and toss to combine.

3. Cover and refrigerate for at least 2 hours to allow the flavors to blend.

Three-Bean Salad

SERVES 8 / PREP TIME: 15 MINUTES, PLUS 2 HOURS TO MARINATE

This salad comes together easily and quickly because it uses canned beans. Be sure to drain the beans thoroughly: Dump them in a colander, give them a good rinse, and let them drain in the sink before adding them to the salad. You can substitute any type of beans you enjoy in this salad, or even replace some of the beans with cooked lentils.

Technique tip: *To quickly mince garlic cloves, put them through a garlic press. Press the garlic directly over the vinaigrette bowl so any juice that comes out of the garlic will flavor the vinaigrette.*

1 (14-ounce) can chickpeas, drained

1 (14-ounce) can green beans, drained

1 (14-ounce) can kidney beans, drained

3 scallions, chopped

¼ cup extra-virgin olive oil

½ cup apple cider vinegar

2 garlic cloves, minced

1 tablespoon shallot, finely minced

1 teaspoon Dijon mustard

Zest of ½ lemon

½ teaspoon sea salt

¼ teaspoon freshly ground black pepper

Dash of cayenne

Nut-free
Vegan

REPAIR

Snacks

PER SERVING
CALORIES: 295
CARBS: 41G
FAT: 10G
PROTEIN: 14G
SUGAR: 6G

1. In a large bowl, combine the chickpeas, green beans, kidney beans, and scallions.

2. In a small bowl, whisk together the olive oil, apple cider vinegar, garlic, shallot, mustard, lemon zest, salt, pepper, and cayenne until well emulsified. Pour over the beans.

3. Allow the salad to marinate for 2 hours in the refrigerator so the flavors blend.

Baked Sweet Potato Crisps

SERVES 4 / PREP TIME: 10 MINUTES / COOK TIME: 25 MINUTES

These tasty chips are delicious by themselves and also pair well with dips. You can make a big batch and keep them at room temperature in a tightly sealed container for up to a week. You'll need to slice the potatoes very thinly to make the chips. If you have a mandoline, set it to cut ¼-inch slices. You can also use a food processor, or just slice very carefully with a knife.

Substitution tip: *While this recipe calls for thyme to season the chips, you can also use chopped fresh rosemary, lemon thyme, or chopped fresh chives.*

Nut-free
Paleo-friendly
Vegan

REPAIR

Snacks

PER SERVING
CALORIES: 196
CARBS: 32G
FAT: 7G
PROTEIN: 2G
SUGAR: 1G

2 sweet potatoes, peeled and cut into ¼-inch slices
2 tablespoons olive oil
2 tablespoons chopped fresh thyme
1 teaspoon sea salt

1. Preheat the oven to 375°F. Line a large baking sheet with parchment paper.

2. In a large bowl, toss the sweet potatoes with the olive oil, thyme, and sea salt.

3. Put the potatoes in a single layer on the baking sheet.

4. Bake for 20 to 25 minutes, flipping the chips after 10 minutes. The chips are done when they begin to brown.

Chickpea and Zucchini Hummus

SERVES 6 / PREP TIME: 10 MINUTES / COOK TIME: 15 MINUTES

Serve this hummus with the Baked Sweet Potato Crisps (page 82). It also tastes delicious with cut-up vegetables, such as sweet bell peppers, celery, carrots, or jicama. The hummus doesn't freeze well, but it will keep in the refrigerator for three to five days. Allow the roasted zucchini to fully cool before adding to the hummus.

1 large zucchini, sliced
4 tablespoons extra-virgin olive oil, divided
2 garlic cloves, crushed through a garlic press
1 cup canned chickpeas, drained
Juice of 1 lemon
2 tablespoons chopped fresh flat-leaf parsley
Sea salt

1. Preheat the oven to 350°F.
2. In a large bowl, toss the zucchini slices with 2 tablespoons olive oil.
3. Put the zucchini on a large baking sheet, and roast until soft, 10 to 15 minutes.
4. Allow the zucchini to cool completely before continuing.
5. In the bowl of a food processor fitted with a metal chopping blade or in a blender, combine the cooled zucchini, the remaining 2 tablespoons olive oil, garlic, chickpeas, lemon juice, and parsley. Process until the hummus is smooth, about 1 minute.
6. Taste and season with sea salt.

Nut-free
Vegan

REPAIR

Snacks

PER SERVING
CALORIES: 212
CARBS: 22G
FAT: 11G
PROTEIN: 7G
SUGAR: 5G

Pumpkin Dip

SERVES 6 / PREP TIME: 5 MINUTES / COOK TIME: 15 MINUTES

The secret ingredient in this savory pumpkin dip is Chinese five-spice powder. You can find this flavorful spice blend in the spice aisle of the grocery store. It adds a little sweet, a little savory, and a little heat to make the flavors of this dip complex. The smoked paprika adds an extra layer of sweet and smoky flavors. Serve the dip with wheat-free crackers.

Technique tip: *If fresh butternut squash is available, you can use it in place of the pumpkin in this recipe. Peel and cut the squash into cubes and toss with olive oil. Roast in a preheated 400°F oven until tender, about 20 minutes. Then purée the squash in a food processor or blender, and add to the recipe in place of the pumpkin in step 3.*

**Nut-free
Paleo-friendly
Vegan**

REPAIR

Snacks

PER SERVING
CALORIES: 50
CARBS: 7G
FAT: 3G
PROTEIN: 1G
SUGAR: 3G

1 tablespoon olive oil

½ red onion, chopped

2 garlic cloves, minced

1 teaspoon smoked paprika

1 teaspoon Chinese five-spice powder

1 tablespoon water

1 (15-ounce) can unsweetened pumpkin purée

1. In a large sauté pan, heat the olive oil over medium-high heat until it shimmers. Add the onion and cook until soft, about 5 minutes. Add the garlic and cook, stirring constantly, until it is fragrant, about 30 seconds.

2. Add the paprika and Chinese five-spice powder, and cook, stirring constantly, until the spices are fragrant, about 1 minute.

3. Reduce the heat to low. Stir in the water and the pumpkin. Cook, stirring frequently, for 5 minutes. Serve warm or chilled.

Black Bean and Pineapple Salsa with Corn Chips

SERVES 4 / PREP TIME: 15 MINUTES / COOK TIME: 4 MINUTES

Pineapple contains bromelain, an enzyme that helps break down and digest protein. Here, pineapple makes the beans easier to digest. You can replace the pineapple with mango or papaya for a twist on this salsa.

4 corn tortillas, cut into wedges

Nonstick cooking spray

1 (15-ounce) can black beans, rinsed and drained

1 (15-ounce) can unsweetened pineapple chunks, drained

½ cup halved cherry tomatoes

½ red onion, diced

¼ cup chopped fresh cilantro

Juice of 1 lime

½ teaspoon cayenne pepper

½ teaspoon ground coriander

½ teaspoon ground cumin

1. Preheat the oven to 400°F.

2. Place the tortilla wedges in a single layer on a baking sheet, and lightly spray them with cooking spray. Bake until the wedges begin to crisp and brown, about 4 minutes.

3. In a medium bowl, combine the beans, pineapple, tomatoes, onion, cilantro, lime juice, cayenne, coriander, and cumin.

4. Serve the salsa with the warm tortilla chips.

Nut-free
Vegan

REPAIR

Snacks

PER SERVING
CALORIES: 214
CARBS: 43G
FAT: 2G
PROTEIN: 9G
SUGAR: 11G

Mediterranean White Bean Dip with Vegetables

SERVES 8 / PREP TIME: 10 MINUTES

This flavorful dip uses cannellini beans as a backdrop for delicious Mediterranean flavors. You can serve the dip with slices of other vegetables, such as zucchini, cucumber, or red bell pepper. It also makes a delicious filling when wrapped in lettuce, spinach, or kale.

Substitution tip: *You can replace the white beans with chickpeas or pinto beans if you can't find the cannellini. Any other white beans will work well, too.*

Nut-free
Vegan

REPAIR

Snacks

PER SERVING
CALORIES: 153
CARBS: 31G
FAT: 1G
PROTEIN: 5G
SUGAR: 2G

1 (15-ounce) can cannellini beans, rinsed and drained

Juice of 1 lemon

½ teaspoon freshly grated lemon zest

¼ cup chopped fresh flat-leaf parsley

1 garlic clove, finely minced

1 teaspoon dried oregano, crumbled

1 teaspoon ground cumin

1 (6-ounce) package rice crackers

15 celery sticks

15 baby carrots

1. In a food processor or a blender, combine the cannellini beans, lemon juice, lemon zest, parsley, garlic, oregano, and cumin.

2. Process until the mixture is smooth, 1 to 2 minutes.

3. Serve the dip with the crackers, celery, and carrots.

Crispy Toasts with Tomato Basil Bruschetta

SERVES 4 / PREP TIME: 15 MINUTES, PLUS 2 HOURS TO MARINATE

This recipe is especially delicious in the summer, when tomatoes, garlic, and basil are in season at your local farmers' market. While any variety of tomato will work, sweet heirloom tomatoes are particularly delicious. You can also substitute halved cherry tomatoes. For best results with the toast, select a whole-grain or multigrain gluten-free bread.

Technique tip: *To chiffonade basil, you will need a very sharp chef's knife. Stack several large fresh basil leaves and roll them into a tight roll. Slice into very thin strips to create a chiffonade.*

2 large ripe tomatoes, chopped

2 tablespoons balsamic vinegar

1 tablespoon extra-virgin olive oil

2 garlic cloves, finely minced

6 large fresh basil leaves, cut in a chiffonade

¼ teaspoon sea salt

¼ teaspoon freshly ground black pepper

4 slices whole-grain or multigrain gluten-free bread, toasted

1 large garlic clove, halved lengthwise

1. In a medium bowl, combine the tomatoes, vinegar, olive oil, minced garlic, basil, salt, and pepper.

2. Cover and marinate at room temperature for 2 hours to allow the flavors to blend.

3. Rub each slice of toast with the cut halves of the garlic clove.

4. Cut each slice of toast into 4 pieces.

5. Serve the toast topped with the tomato mixture.

Nut-free
Vegan

REPAIR

Snacks

PER SERVING
CALORIES: 121
CARBS: 18G
FAT: 5G
PROTEIN: 3G
SUGAR: 4G

Pecan Granola Bars

SERVES 12 / PREP TIME: 10 MINUTES / COOK TIME: 25 MINUTES

Granola contains oats, which are often cross-contaminated with gluten during processing. To be sure you're not adding unwanted gluten, buy certified gluten-free granola. Also, choose a granola that doesn't contain sugar; instead, look for one that has been sweetened with pure maple syrup or honey.

Ingredient tip: *Make sure the syrup you use is pure maple syrup, not pancake syrup. Pancake syrup is often made with refined sugars such as high-fructose corn syrup or white sugar, while pure maple syrup is made from boiling the sap of maple trees—with nothing added.*

Vegetarian

REPAIR

Snacks

PER SERVING
CALORIES: 144
CARBS: 12G
FAT: 10G
PROTEIN: 3G
SUGAR: 3G

2 tablespoons pure maple syrup

1 egg white, beaten

2 teaspoons coconut oil, melted

½ teaspoon vanilla extract

½ teaspoon ground cinnamon

2 cups gluten-free granola

¼ cup chopped pecans

1. Preheat the oven to 325°F. Line a 9-inch-square baking pan with parchment paper.

2. In a large bowl, whisk together the syrup, egg white, coconut oil, vanilla, and cinnamon until well combined.

3. Stir in the granola and pecans.

4. Press the mixture into the prepared pan.

5. Bake until the mixture is browned, about 25 minutes.

6. Allow the granola bars to cool on a wire rack. When cooled, cut into 12 pieces.

Eggplant and Artichoke Casserole

SERVES 8 / PREP TIME: 10 MINUTES / COOK TIME: 30 MINUTES

This hearty casserole is warming and delicious. It creates a layered dish, similar to lasagna. You can cook the casserole ahead of time and then cut it into portions and refrigerate, tightly sealed, for up to five days. Reheat it in the microwave.

Ingredient tip: *Eggplant can be bitter and watery. To remove the bitterness and make it less watery when you cook it, slice the eggplant and place the slices in a colander. Salt the slices, and place the colander in the sink for half an hour. The salt will draw out the water and bitterness. Then wipe the eggplant completely clean of salt with a paper towel, and use as directed in the recipe.*

1½ cups sugar-free tomato sauce, divided

12 soft corn tortillas, divided

2 tablespoons olive oil, divided

1 medium eggplant, thinly sliced

½ teaspoon salt, divided

½ teaspoon freshly ground black pepper, divided

1 small zucchini, thinly sliced

1 (15-ounce) can artichoke hearts, drained

1 teaspoon dried oregano

1 teaspoon dried basil

½ teaspoon dried marjoram

Nut-free
Vegan

REPAIR

Dinner

PER SERVING
CALORIES: 165
CARBS: 27G
FAT: 5G
PROTEIN: 4G
SUGAR: 3G

1. Preheat the oven to 350°F.

2. Pour ¾ cup tomato sauce into a nonstick or ceramic lasagna pan or casserole dish to cover the bottom. Cover the tomato sauce with 6 of the corn tortillas, cutting the tortillas so they fit in a single layer.

3. In a large nonstick skillet over medium-high heat, heat 1 tablespoon olive oil. Add the eggplant in a single layer. Sprinkle it with ¼ teaspoon salt and ¼ teaspoon pepper.

4. Sauté until the eggplant begins to soften, about 3 minutes. Flip and repeat cooking on the other side, moving the cooked pieces onto the tortillas in the lasagna pan in a single layer. »

Eggplant and Artichoke Casserole *continued*

5. Add the remaining 1 tablespoon olive oil to the skillet over medium-high heat. Add the zucchini slices to the skillet in a single layer, and sprinkle them with the remaining ¼ teaspoon salt and ¼ teaspoon pepper. Cook, stirring occasionally, until the zucchini softens, about 4 minutes. Layer the cooked zucchini on top of the eggplant in the lasagna pan.

6. Arrange the artichoke hearts on top of the zucchini in the lasagna pan. Sprinkle the vegetables with the oregano, basil, and marjoram. Top with the remaining 6 corn tortillas, again cutting them to fit in a single layer. Spoon the remaining ¾ cup tomato sauce over the casserole.

7. Bake until heated through, about 20 minutes.

Quinoa Pasta with Sautéed Mushrooms

SERVES: 4 / PREP TIME: 15 MINUTES / COOK TIME: 20 MINUTES

Many grocery stores now carry pasta made from the supergrain quinoa, which is high in protein. When combined with a rich mushroom topping, it creates a delicious meal with earthy and tasty flavors. While the recipe calls for crimini mushrooms, you can also use any seasonal mushrooms that are available, such as shiitake, oyster, or chanterelle.

8 ounces dry quinoa pasta, any shape

1 tablespoon extra-virgin olive oil

1 onion, minced

1 pound crimini mushrooms, stemmed and sliced

2 garlic cloves, minced

2 teaspoons chopped fresh thyme

½ cup low-sodium chicken broth

Sea salt

Freshly ground black pepper

Nut-free
Vegan

REPAIR

Dinner

PER SERVING
CALORIES: 236
CARBS: 39G
FAT: 5G
PROTEIN: 11G
SUGAR: 3G

1. Prepare the pasta according to the package instructions, and drain.

2. While the pasta cooks, heat the olive oil in a large sauté pan over medium-high heat until it shimmers.

3. Add the onion and cook, stirring occasionally, until it is soft, about 5 minutes.

4. Add the mushrooms and cook, stirring occasionally, until they brown and release their liquid, about 7 minutes.

5. Add the garlic and cook, stirring constantly, until it is fragrant, about 30 seconds.

6. Add the thyme and broth, scraping any browned bits from the bottom of the pan with the spoon. Simmer until the broth reduces by half, 4 to 5 minutes.

7. Season with salt and pepper. Toss with the cooked pasta and serve immediately.

Brown Rice Bowl with Vegetables

SERVES 4 / PREP TIME: 10 MINUTES / COOK TIME: 15 MINUTES

Use instant or precooked brown rice for this dish. You can find precooked brown rice in the freezer or rice section of the supermarket. Avoid the sugar found in store-bought sriracha sauce by preparing the Do-It-Yourself Sriracha recipe (page 37) in advance. If you're short on time, look for sugar-free sriracha at your local grocery store.

Nut-free
Vegan

REPAIR

Dinner

PER SERVING
CALORIES: 331
CARBS: 49G
FAT: 12G
PROTEIN: 8G
SUGAR: 4G

1 tablespoon olive oil

2 teaspoons sesame oil

2 tablespoons grated fresh ginger

1 medium onion, chopped

6 scallions, chopped

1 green bell pepper, seeded and chopped

1 carrot, peeled and sliced

2 garlic cloves, minced

½ cup low-sodium vegetable broth

2 tablespoons gluten-free soy sauce

½ teaspoon Do-It-Yourself Sriracha

2 cups cooked brown rice

4 tablespoons sesame seeds, divided

1. In a large sauté pan or wok, heat the olive oil, sesame oil, and ginger over medium-high heat until the oil shimmers.

2. Add the chopped onion, scallions, bell pepper, and carrot. Cook, stirring frequently, until the vegetables are crisp-tender, about 5 minutes.

3. Add the garlic and cook until it is fragrant, about 30 seconds. Add the broth, soy sauce, and sriracha, scraping any browned bits from the bottom of the pan with the spoon.

4. Reduce the heat to medium, and simmer until the sauce thickens slightly, about 4 minutes.

5. Stir in the rice and cook, stirring constantly, until the rice heats through, about 4 minutes.

6. Divide the mixture among 4 bowls. Top each serving with 1 tablespoon sesame seeds, and serve.

Slow Cooker Wild Rice with Mushrooms and Dried Cranberries

SERVES 4 / PREP TIME: 10 MINUTES / COOK TIME: 6 HOURS IN A SLOW COOKER

Wild rice isn't really rice at all. It's actually a grass. It takes about 40 minutes to cook on the stovetop or about 6 hours in a slow cooker. Prepare this satisfying meal in a slow cooker, and it will be ready to go at dinnertime with minimal effort.

1½ cups wild rice

2 (14-ounce) cans low-sodium vegetable broth

8 ounces crimini mushrooms, stemmed and sliced

1 teaspoon dried thyme

½ teaspoon dried sage

½ teaspoon fine sea salt

¼ teaspoon freshly ground black pepper

1 cup dried unsweetened cranberries

½ cup coarsely chopped toasted walnuts

1. In a slow cooker, combine the rice, broth, mushrooms, thyme, sage, salt, and pepper. Cover and set on low.

2. Cook until the rice softens, about 6 hours.

3. Stir in the dried cranberries and walnuts. Allow them to heat through, and serve.

Vegan

REPAIR

Dinner

PER SERVING
CALORIES: 400
CARBS: 51G
FAT: 11G
PROTEIN: 14G
SUGAR: 3G

BBQ Baked Beans and Greens

SERVES 4 / PREP TIME: 10 MINUTES / COOK TIME: 35 MINUTES

This recipe uses homemade barbecue sauce, which you can use in other recipes as well. Most commercial barbecue sauce has added sugar or high-fructose corn syrup, so it's best to make your own. Two ingredients give homemade barbecue sauce a smoky flavor: smoked paprika and liquid smoke. Liquid smoke can be quite strong—a little goes a long way.

Ingredient tip: *You can make the barbecue sauce and save it, tightly covered, in the refrigerator for up to two weeks. The barbecue sauce is low in carbs and fat, so it will work in all stages of this diet.*

Nut-free
Vegan

REPAIR

Dinner

PER SERVING
CALORIES: 327
CARBS: 49G
FAT: 8G
PROTEIN: 16G
SUGAR: 5G

2 tablespoons olive oil, divided

½ red onion, minced

2 garlic cloves, minced

2 tablespoons tomato paste

½ cup apple cider vinegar

½ cup sugar-free tomato sauce

1 tablespoon smoked paprika

1 tablespoon chili powder

1 tablespoon Dijon mustard

¼ teaspoon liquid smoke

½ teaspoon salt, divided

½ teaspoons freshly ground black pepper

¼ teaspoon ground cloves

Dash cayenne pepper

2 (15-ounce) cans navy beans, rinsed and drained

1 medium onion, chopped

10 ounces fresh spinach

2 tablespoons low-sodium vegetable broth

1. In a large saucepan, heat 1 tablespoon olive oil over medium-high heat until it shimmers. Add the red onion and cook until it softens and begins to brown, about 6 minutes. Add the garlic and cook until it is fragrant, about 30 seconds.

2. Add the tomato paste and cook, stirring constantly, until the tomato paste begins to brown, about 4 minutes.

3. Add the vinegar and stir to combine, scraping any browned bits from the bottom of the pan the spoon.

4. Stir in the tomato sauce, smoked paprika, chili powder, mustard, liquid smoke, ¼ teaspoon salt, black pepper, cloves, and cayenne. Bring to a simmer, and allow the flavors to blend and the sauce to thicken slightly, about 8 minutes.

5. Add the beans and reduce the heat to low. Simmer until the beans warm through, about 5 minutes more.

6. Meanwhile, in a medium sauté pan, heat the remaining 1 tablespoon olive oil over medium-high heat until it shimmers. Add the onion and cook until it is soft, about 4 minutes.

7. Add the spinach and remaining ¼ teaspoon salt, and cook for 2 minutes. Add the broth and cook just until the spinach wilts, about 3 more minutes.

8. Serve the beans with a side of the greens.

REPAIR

Dinner

Hearty Potato-Leek Soup

SERVES 4 / PREP TIME: 15 MINUTES / COOK TIME: 35 MINUTES

Potato and leeks are a classic combination that makes a creamy, hearty soup with a big flavor. Choose a starchy potato such as Russet or a baking potato for this soup. Yukon Gold potatoes also work well. Because leeks often have dirt between their layers, be sure to thoroughly clean them by swishing them around in a large bowl of water and repeating the process until no dirt settles to the bottom of the bowl.

Substitution tip: *To make this soup Paleo-friendly, or to just change flavor profiles, use sweet potatoes in place of the potatoes.*

Nut-free

REPAIR

Dinner

PER SERVING
CALORIES: 371
CARBS: 69G
FAT: 8G
PROTEIN: 8G
SUGAR: 8G

2 tablespoons olive oil

3 leeks, white part only, cleaned and sliced

6 cups low-sodium chicken broth

4 large potatoes, peeled and cut into ½-inch cubes

1 teaspoon dried thyme

Sea salt

Freshly ground black pepper

1. In a large pot, heat the olive oil over medium-high heat until it shimmers. Add the leeks and cook, stirring occasionally, until they begin to soften, about 5 minutes.

2. Add the broth, potatoes, and thyme. Bring the soup to a boil; then reduce the heat to medium and cook until the potatoes and leeks are tender, about 20 minutes.

3. Carefully transfer the hot soup in batches to a blender or food processor. Put the lid on, leaving the spout at the top open so steam can escape. Fold a towel several times, and place it on top of the blender or food processor. Put your hand on top of the towel to hold the lid in place. Blend, pausing to let steam escape, until the soup is smooth, about 1 to 2 minutes.

4. Season with salt and pepper.

Baked Sweet Potato with Pineapple

SERVES 4 / PREP TIME: 5 MINUTES / COOK TIME: 50 MINUTES

This recipe is so easy, you can make it in a toaster oven. It is also extremely satisfying. Sweet potatoes are loaded with fiber and nutrients, and have a wonderful, earthy flavor. Serve with a side of steamed or roasted broccoli.

4 sweet potatoes
Fine sea salt
Freshly ground black pepper
1 (15-ounce) can sugar-free crushed pineapple, drained

1. Preheat the oven to 350°F.

2. Score the sweet potatoes with a small X on top, and place them in a baking pan large enough to hold them in a single layer.

3. Bake until soft, about 50 minutes.

4. Cut open the potatoes, and season them with salt and pepper. Spoon some of the crushed pineapple onto each potato.

Nut-free
Paleo-friendly
Vegan

REPAIR

Dinner

PER SERVING
CALORIES: 230
CARBS: 56G
FAT: 0G
PROTEIN: 3G
SUGAR: 11G

Halibut with Mango and Watercress Salad

SERVES 4 / PREP TIME: 10 MINUTES / COOK TIME: 10 MINUTES

Swapping cod for halibut makes this dish more approachable for everyday dining. Both halibut and cod should be cooked all the way through and not to medium-rare. You can also use sea scallops or shrimp in place of the fish.

2 teaspoons ground coriander, divided

1 pound halibut, cut into 4 equal pieces

Fine sea salt

Freshly ground black pepper

2 ripe mangos, peeled, pitted, and diced

¼ cup chopped fresh cilantro

1 red jalapeño pepper, seeded and minced

Zest and juice of 1 lime

1 bunch watercress, trimmed

Nut-free
Paleo-friendly

REPAIR

Dinner

PER SERVING
CALORIES: 234
CARBS: 18G
FAT: 4G
PROTEIN: 31G
SUGAR: 16G

1. Preheat the oven to 450°F. Line a baking sheet with parchment paper.

2. Sprinkle 1 teaspoon coriander evenly over both sides of the halibut. Season with salt and pepper.

3. Put the halibut on the prepared baking sheet, and bake until it is juicy and flakes when pressed, 8 to 12 minutes.

4. Meanwhile, in a medium bowl, toss together the mangos, cilantro, jalapeño, lime zest, lime juice, ¼ teaspoon sea salt, and the remaining 1 teaspoon coriander. Add the watercress to the bowl, and toss with the dressing.

5. Serve the salad with the halibut.

Baked Red Snapper with Summer Fruit

SERVES 4 / PREP TIME: 10 MINUTES / COOK TIME: 20 MINUTES

Tomatoes are at their best in late summer, and pair nicely with watermelon. This recipe works especially well with locally grown sweet heirloom tomatoes. Look for them at the farmers' market. For a change, swap the watermelon for pitted fresh cherries or the blueberries for raspberries.

Nonstick cooking spray
1 cup blueberries
1 cup chopped watermelon
½ cup chopped fresh tomatoes
¼ cup fresh mint leaves, slivered
¼ cup fresh basil leaves, slivered
½ teaspoon salt, divided
4 (4-ounce) red snapper fillets
½ teaspoon ground cumin
⅛ teaspoon white pepper
1 lemon, thinly sliced

1. Preheat the oven to 400°F. Spray a 9-by-9-inch square glass baking dish with nonstick cooking spray and set it aside.

2. In a medium bowl, combine the blueberries, watermelon, tomatoes, mint, basil, and ¼ teaspoon salt. Mix well and set aside.

3. Arrange the fillets in the prepared pan. Sprinkle with the cumin, white pepper, and the remaining ¼ teaspoon salt. Top with the lemon slices.

4. Bake until the fish is opaque and its flesh flakes when tested with fork, 15 to 20 minutes.

5. Serve topped with the fruit salsa.

Nut-free
Paleo-friendly

REPAIR

Dinner

PER SERVING
CALORIES: 184
CARBS: 10G
FAT: 2G
PROTEIN: 31G
SUGAR: 6G

Citrus-Ginger Salmon

SERVES 4 / PREP TIME: 30 MINUTES (INCLUDES MARINATING TIME) /
COOK TIME: 10 MINUTES

Most varieties of fish taste great with a bit of citrus. The ginger makes this dish even more special. Serve this no-fail recipe when you have company coming over. You will spend most of the party with your guests, not in the kitchen.

1 navel orange
Zest and juice of 1 lime
1 (2-inch) piece fresh ginger, peeled and finely minced
2 tablespoons olive oil, divided
1 (1-pound) salmon fillet, skin-on
Fine sea salt
Freshly ground black pepper

Nut-free
Paleo-friendly

REPAIR

Dinner

PER SERVING
CALORIES: 192
CARBS: 5G
FAT: 9G
PROTEIN: 24G
SUGAR: 4G

1. Zest the orange into a pie plate and set aside. Peel the orange, and slice it into rounds. Put the orange slices in a small bowl.

2. Zest the lime into the pie plate with the orange zest. Cut the lime in half, and squeeze all of its juice into the pie plate.

3. Whisk the ginger and 1 tablespoon olive oil into the pie plate mixture.

4. Sprinkle the salmon with salt and pepper; then place it, flesh-side down, in the marinade. Marinate in the refrigerator for 20 minutes.

5. In a cast iron pan, heat the remaining 1 tablespoon olive oil over medium-high heat until it shimmers. Place the fish, skin-side down, in the pan. Sear until the skin turns brown and crispy, about 2 minutes. Carefully turn the fish over, and cook until it is medium-rare, about 6 more minutes.

6. Serve with the orange slices.

Cioppino

SERVES 8 / PREP TIME: 10 MINUTES / COOK TIME: 35 MINUTES

This seafood stew pairs delicious fish and shellfish with fragrant fennel, tomatoes, onions, and garlic for a classic Italian flavor profile. Carefully pick over and clean the clams and mussels before using them, and be sure to discard any that are cracked or open. Serve the stew hot, with bowls on the side to discard clam and mussel shells.

Substitution tip: *You can replace the halibut in this recipe with any firm-fleshed fish, such as cod or salmon. If you don't like the flavor of fennel, you can substitute 2 sliced celery ribs.*

2 tablespoons olive oil

2 medium sweet onions, chopped

1 large fennel bulb, thinly sliced

4 garlic cloves, minced

1 (8-ounce) bottle clam juice

6 cups low-sodium chicken broth

2 (15-ounce) cans crushed tomatoes, with juice

1 bay leaf

1 teaspoon dried thyme

1 teaspoon dried oregano

½ teaspoon red pepper flakes

12 Manila clams

12 mussels

1½ pounds uncooked large shrimp, peeled and deveined

1 pound halibut fillets, cut into 1-inch chunks

¼ cup minced fresh flat-leaf parsley

Fine sea salt

Freshly ground black pepper

Nut-free

REPAIR

Dinner

PER SERVING
CALORIES: 307
CARBS: 21G
FAT: 6G
PROTEIN: 42G
SUGAR: 8G

1. In a large stockpot, heat the olive oil over medium-high heat until it shimmers. Add the onions and fennel, and cook, stirring occasionally, until the vegetables are soft and begin to brown, about 5 minutes. Add the garlic and cook until it is fragrant, about 30 seconds. »

Cioppino *continued*

2. Add the clam juice, using the spoon to scrape any browned bits from the bottom of the pot. Add the broth, crushed tomatoes and their juice, bay leaf, thyme, oregano, and red pepper flakes. Cover and simmer until the flavors combine, about 20 minutes.

3. Stir in the clams, mussels, shrimp, and halibut. Cover and simmer until the clams and mussels open and the fish cooks through, 5 to 7 minutes. Discard any clams or mussels that did not open.

4. Stir in the parsley. Season with salt and pepper.

REPAIR

Dinner

Mussels in Tomato Sauce

SERVES 4 / PREP TIME: 10 MINUTES / COOK TIME: 40 MINUTES

Shellfish pairs well with tomato sauce. Serve the mussels in a bowl with the tomato sauce spooned over the top, and offer a toasted gluten-free crusty bread to dip in the sauce. Be sure to provide extra bowls for the discarded mussel shells.

Ingredient tip: *To clean the mussels, look them over and discard any with shells that are broken, cracked, open, or chipped. Soak the mussels in cold water just before cooking to remove any sand, and then remove the mussel beards by pulling the thin seaweed-like thread away from the mussel until it detaches.*

2 tablespoons olive oil

1 onion, finely chopped

3 garlic cloves, minced

2 tablespoons chopped fresh thyme

¾ cup clam juice

1 (28-ounce) can peeled and diced tomatoes, juice reserved

2 pounds mussels

Fine sea salt

Freshly ground black pepper

2 tablespoons chopped fresh flat-leaf parsley

Nut-free
Paleo-friendly

REPAIR

Dinner

PER SERVING
CALORIES: 328
CARBS: 23G
FAT: 12G
PROTEIN: 29G
SUGAR: 8G

1. In a deep sauté pan, heat the olive oil over medium-high heat until it shimmers. Add the onion and sauté until it softens and begins to brown, about 8 minutes.

2. Stir in the garlic and thyme, and cook until they are fragrant, about 30 seconds.

3. Add the clam juice. Bring the liquid to a simmer, and cook for 5 minutes. Add the tomatoes. Cover and let simmer for 20 minutes.

4. Add the mussels and stir to combine. If the tomatoes have reduced too far to evenly coat the mussels, add the reserved tomato liquid, ¼ cup at a time, until the consistency is saucy.

5. Cook the mussels, stirring occasionally, until the shells open, 4 to 5 minutes. Discard any mussels that did not open.

6. Season with salt and pepper, sprinkle with parsley, and serve.

Baked Scallops with Mango Salsa

SERVES 4 / PREP TIME: 15 MINUTES / COOK TIME: 20 MINUTES

A spicy, fruity salsa complements the sweetness of large sea scallops perfectly. Select large, fresh scallops with a pearly sheen that do not smell fishy, or choose frozen sea scallops. Pick mangos that yield lightly to pressure without being mushy.

Substitution tip: *Mango salsa also tastes great with other white fish, such as baked cod or grilled halibut. For a smokier flavor in this dish, thread the scallops on skewers and cook them on the grill until they are opaque, about 15 minutes.*

Nut-free
Paleo-friendly

REPAIR

Dinner

PER SERVING
CALORIES: 226
CARBS: 23G
FAT: 8G
PROTEIN: 16G
SUGAR: 17G

12 large sea scallops

2 tablespoons olive oil

Fine sea salt

Freshly ground black pepper

2 mangos, peeled and diced

1 red onion, diced

1 jalapeño pepper, seeded and minced

1 garlic clove, minced

¼ cup chopped fresh cilantro

Juice of 1 lime

1. Preheat the oven to 400°F.

2. In a large bowl, toss the scallops with the olive oil. Place the scallops in a baking pan, and season them with salt and pepper.

3. Bake the scallops until they are firm and opaque, about 20 minutes.

4. Meanwhile, in a small bowl combine the mangos, onion, jalapeño, garlic, cilantro, and lime juice. Allow the salsa to sit so the flavors blend while the scallops cook.

5. Serve the scallops topped with the mango salsa.

Shrimp with Tropical Fruit Salsa

SERVES 4 / PREP TIME: 15 MINUTES / COOK TIME: 2 MINUTES

Fresh papaya from Hawaii kicks this dish up a notch. If you can't find fresh pineapple, use unsweetened canned pineapple instead.

Ingredient tip: *Make the salsa ahead of time and allow it to sit, refrigerated, overnight. This will save you time in the final preparation, and it also allows the flavors to blend.*

2 bananas, cut into ¼-inch pieces

1 large papaya, peeled and cut into ¼-inch chunks

1 cup fresh pineapple chunks

7 ounces canned hearts of palm, drained and sliced

½ cup chopped fresh cilantro

⅓ cup chopped red onion

Zest and juice of 1 lime

¼ teaspoon fine sea salt

1 pound uncooked shrimp, peeled and deveined

2 teaspoons Old Bay seasoning

1 tablespoon olive oil

Nut-free
Paleo-friendly

REPAIR

Dinner

PER SERVING
CALORIES: 309
CARBS: 37G
FAT: 6G
PROTEIN: 29G
SUGAR: 21G

1. In a large bowl, toss together the bananas, papaya, pineapple, hearts of palm, cilantro, onion, lime zest, lime juice, and salt. Set aside.

2. In a medium bowl, toss the shrimp with the Old Bay seasoning.

3. In a cast iron pan, heat the olive oil over medium-high heat until it shimmers. Add the shrimp and sear it, 1 minute per side, until pink and just cooked through. Remove from the heat.

4. Serve with the salsa.

Black Bean Soup with Ground Turkey and Sweet Potatoes

SERVES 4 / PREP TIME: 10 MINUTES / COOK TIME: 30 MINUTES

If you make a big batch of this soup, you can freeze half in individual portions for lunches or quick dinners during the week. Measure 1-cup servings into zip-top bags, and store in the freezer for up to one year.

2 tablespoons olive oil, divided

½ pound ground turkey breast

1 small onion, chopped

3 cups low-sodium chicken broth

1 large sweet potato, peeled and cut into ½-inch chunks

1 teaspoon ground coriander

1 teaspoon ground cumin

½ teaspoon cayenne pepper

¼ teaspoon fine sea salt

2 (15-ounce) cans black beans, rinsed and drained

Juice of 1 lime

2 tablespoons chopped fresh cilantro

Nut-free

REPAIR

Dinner

PER SERVING
CALORIES: 422
CARBS: 44G
FAT: 13G
PROTEIN: 31G
SUGAR: 4G

1. In a large pot, heat 1 tablespoon olive oil over medium-high heat until it shimmers. Add the ground turkey and cook, stirring frequently until it is cooked through, about 5 minutes. Remove to a bowl and set aside.

2. Add the remaining 1 tablespoon olive oil and the onion to the pot. Cook, stirring often, until the onion is soft and beginning to brown, about 6 minutes.

3. Add the broth, sweet potato, coriander, cumin, cayenne, and salt.

4. Turn the heat to high, and bring the soup to a low boil. Cover and reduce the heat to medium-low. Cook until the sweet potato is tender, about 15 minutes.

5. Add the black beans and reserved turkey. Bring to a simmer.

6. Remove from the heat, and stir in the lime juice and cilantro just before serving.

Chicken Pad Thai

SERVES 4 / PREP TIME: 20 MINUTES / COOK TIME: 20 MINUTES

Pad Thai gets its classic sweet and sour taste from tamarind paste and salty fish sauce. Fish sauce is made from fermented fish and sea salt, and tastes a lot better than it sounds. You can find both in Asian markets or in the international food aisle of your grocery store. Prepare the Do-It-Yourself Sriracha recipe (page 37) in advance, or look for sugar-free sriracha sauce.

Serving tip: *Garnish your pad Thai with grated raw vegetables, such as carrots or cabbage, or with fresh bean sprouts and chopped peanuts.*

1½ tablespoons tamarind paste

2 tablespoons fish sauce

¼ teaspoon Do-It-Yourself Sriracha

1 packet stevia

8 ounces Thai rice noodles

2 tablespoons coconut oil

2 (5-ounce) boneless, skinless chicken breasts, thinly sliced

3 garlic cloves, finely minced

¼ teaspoon red pepper flakes

Nut-free

REPAIR

Dinner

PER SERVING
CALORIES: 416
CARBS: 52G
FAT: 12G
PROTEIN: 23G
SUGAR: 2G

1. In a small bowl, whisk together the tamarind paste, fish sauce, sriracha, and stevia. Set aside.

2. Fill a large pot with very hot water. Add the rice noodles, and cover the pot. Soak the noodles until they are al dente, usually about 8 minutes. Check the package directions to ensure the proper soaking time. Drain the noodles.

3. In a large sauté pan, heat the coconut oil over medium-high heat until it shimmers. Add the chicken and sauté, stirring occasionally, until it is cooked through, 7 to 10 minutes.

4. Add the garlic and cook until it is fragrant, about 30 seconds.

5. Add the noodles, red pepper flakes, and tamarind sauce to the pan. Stir to combine well.

Arroz con Pollo

SERVES 4 / PREP TIME: 15 MINUTES / COOK TIME: 30 MINUTES

Arroz con pollo is a classic Latin American dish of chicken and rice. This version has lycopene-rich tomatoes and vitamin A-rich carrots, along with mushrooms and aromatic vegetables, herbs, and spices. The result is a delicious and flavorful dish with a Latin flair. Serve topped with fresh pico de gallo (see Breakfast Tacos, page 151) or chopped fresh cilantro.

2 (5-ounce) boneless, skinless chicken breast halves, cut into slices

Sea salt

Freshly ground black pepper

½ teaspoon smoked paprika

3 tablespoons extra-virgin olive oil, divided

1 onion, chopped

1 carrot, peeled and chopped

1 green bell pepper, chopped

4 garlic cloves, minced

1 cup long-grain white rice

2 cups low-sodium chicken broth

8 ounces mushrooms, sliced

1 (14-ounce) can chopped tomatoes, drained

Nut-free

REPAIR

Dinner

PER SERVING
CALORIES: 476
CARBS: 50G
FAT: 17G
PROTEIN: 29G
SUGAR: 7G

1. Put the chicken in a bowl, and season with salt, pepper, and smoked paprika.

2. In a large pot, heat 2 tablespoons olive oil over medium-high heat until it shimmers. Add the chicken and cook, stirring occasionally, until no longer pink and the juices run clear. Remove the chicken from the pot with a slotted spoon, and set aside on a platter.

3. Add the remaining 1 tablespoon olive oil to the pot. Add the onion, carrot, and bell pepper. Cook, stirring occasionally, until the vegetables are soft, about 5 minutes.

4. Add the garlic and cook, stirring constantly, until it is fragrant, about 30 seconds.

5. Add the rice, broth, mushrooms, and tomatoes, scraping any browned bits from the bottom of the pot with the spoon. Cover and simmer until the rice is cooked, about 20 minutes.

6. Add the chicken and any juices that have collected on the platter to the rice. Stir to reheat the chicken, about 2 to 3 minutes more.

REPAIR

Dinner

Parsnip and Carrot Hash with Pork

SERVES 4 / PREP TIME: 20 MINUTES / COOK TIME: 20 MINUTES

The next time you cook pork, make a little extra so that you can pull together this dish in no time. Parsnips and carrots are naturally sweet, which makes them a perfect accompaniment to pork.

1 cup low-sodium vegetable broth, divided

2 tablespoons apple cider vinegar

2 teaspoons gluten-free soy sauce

2 teaspoons olive oil

2 onions, chopped

4 carrots, peeled and cut into ½-inch dice

4 parsnips, peeled and cut into ½-inch dice

2 large garlic cloves, minced

1 teaspoon minced fresh thyme

¼ teaspoon salt

¼ teaspoon black pepper

1½ cups (about 6 ounces) diced cooked pork tenderloin

¼ cup chopped fresh flat-leaf parsley

Nut-free

REPAIR

Dinner

PER SERVING
CALORIES: 264
CARBS: 37G
FAT: 5G
PROTEIN: 19G
SUGAR: 12G

1. In a small bowl, combine ¼ cup broth, the cider vinegar, and soy sauce and set aside.

2. In a large cast iron skillet, heat the olive oil over medium-high heat until it shimmers. Add the onions, carrots, and parsnips, and cook until the vegetables are browned in spots, 5 to 8 minutes. Add the garlic and thyme, and cook, stirring, until fragrant, about 30 seconds.

3. Stir in the remaining ¾ cup broth, and cook, scraping up any browned bits from the bottom of the pan, until the liquid is absorbed and the vegetables are tender, about 5 minutes. Season with salt and pepper.

4. Stir in the cider vinegar mixture and the pork. Cook until the pork is heated through and the sauce has thickened slightly, about 2 minutes.

5. Stir in the parsley and serve.

Slow Cooker Pork Loin with Apples, Fennel, and Cabbage

SERVES 4 / PREP TIME: 10 MINUTES / COOK TIME: 4 TO 8 HOURS IN A SLOW COOKER

Apples, pork, fennel, and cabbage are a classic fall combination. This recipe is particularly delicious during the fall harvest, when farmers' markets are bursting with freshly picked versions of the fruits and vegetables this recipe calls for. Choose a sweet-tart apple, such as a Honeycrisp or Gala, for this delicious recipe.

Ingredient tip: *Any type of cabbage will work for this recipe. Try green cabbage, Napa cabbage, red cabbage, or even bok choy. Add the cabbage in the last hour of cooking so it has time to soften but doesn't get mushy.*

Nut-free
Paleo-friendly

REPAIR

Dinner

PER SERVING
CALORIES: 397
CARBS: 17G
FAT: 8G
PROTEIN: 61G
SUGAR: 7G

1 apple, cored and cut into thin slices
1 fennel bulb, thinly sliced
1 red onion, thinly sliced
4 garlic cloves, sliced
¼ cup apple cider vinegar
¼ teaspoon ground cinnamon
1 teaspoon garlic powder
1 (2-pound) whole pork tenderloin
Sea salt
Freshly ground black pepper
2 cups shredded cabbage

1. In a slow cooker, combine the apple, fennel, onion, garlic slices, apple cider vinegar, cinnamon, and garlic powder. Stir to combine.

2. Season the pork tenderloin with salt and pepper, and add it to the slow cooker, covering it with the vegetables.

3. Cover and cook on high for about 4 hours or low for about 8 hours.

4. One hour before serving, stir in the cabbage. Cover the slow cooker, and cook for an additional hour.

Pork with Fava Beans and Strawberries

SERVES 4 / PREP TIME: 10 MINUTES, PLUS 30 MINUTES TO 24 HOURS TO MARINATE / COOK TIME: 45 MINUTES

Favas and strawberries come into season at about the same time. If you're using fresh fava beans, the extra effort of shelling them rewards you with the smooth, fresh taste of the bean. You can also buy them already shelled and frozen.

Substitution tip: *If you're not fond of fava beans, you can replace them with any other type of bean, such as lima beans or kidney beans.*

¼ cup plus 3 tablespoons olive oil

⅓ cup apple cider vinegar

1½ teaspoons fine sea salt, divided

1 teaspoon freshly ground black pepper, divided

1 tablespoon chopped fresh rosemary

1 teaspoon chopped fresh thyme

1¼ pounds pork tenderloin

1 tablespoon Dijon mustard

1 pound frozen fava beans

2 cups low-sodium chicken broth

½ onion, coarsely chopped

3 garlic cloves, minced

1 pint strawberries, hulled and halved

REPAIR

Dinner

PER SERVING
CALORIES: 472
CARBS: 33G
FAT: 16G
PROTEIN: 47G
SUGAR: 7G

1. In a large zip-top bag, combine ¼ cup olive oil, vinegar, ¾ teaspoon salt, ½ teaspoon pepper, the rosemary, and thyme. Mix well, and then add the pork, turning to coat all sides. Seal the bag and marinate in the refrigerator for at least 30 minutes or up to 24 hours.

2. Preheat the oven to 375°F.

3. In a large, oven-safe sauté pan, heat the remaining 3 tablespoons olive oil over medium-high heat until it shimmers. Remove the tenderloin from the bag, and discard the marinade. Add the tenderloin to the pan, and sear for 2 minutes on each side. Transfer the tenderloin to a plate, and brush with the mustard.

4. Add the fava beans, broth, onion, garlic, remaining ¾ teaspoon salt, and remaining ½ teaspoon pepper to the pan, using the side of the spoon to scrape up any brown bits. Bring the mixture to a simmer. Return the tenderloin to the pan, nestling it into the beans. Cover the pan and put it in the oven.

5. Roast the pork for 20 minutes or until it reaches an internal temperature of 145°F. Transfer the pork to a carving board, tent with foil, and allow it to rest for 10 minutes.

6. Meanwhile, place the pan of fava beans over medium-high heat, and bring it to a simmer. Cook until the liquid has almost entirely evaporated, about 10 minutes.

7. Thinly slice the pork, and serve with the fava beans and strawberries.

REPAIR

Dinner

Rack of Lamb with Apricot Relish

SERVES 4 / PREP TIME: 20 MINUTES / COOK TIME: 25 MINUTES

The acidity of the apricots in this dish works nicely with the big flavor of lamb, counterbalancing some of lamb's gaminess. To dress this dish up for company, you can purée the apricots and serve them warm as a sauce.

Ingredient tip: *Kosher salt is a flaked salt that clings especially well to food because of its large, irregular grains. It is less dense than table salt, so you need more kosher salt than you do table or sea salt to get the same saltiness. If you don't have kosher salt on hand, you can replace it with ¼ teaspoon sea salt.*

Nut-free
Paleo-friendly

REPAIR

Dinner

PER SERVING
CALORIES: 277
CARBS: 6G
FAT: 17G
PROTEIN: 24G
SUGAR: 3G

1 teaspoon ground cinnamon

¾ teaspoon freshly ground black pepper

¾ teaspoon ground cumin

½ teaspoon ground turmeric

½ teaspoon kosher salt, divided

⅛ teaspoon ground cloves

1 tablespoon plus 1 teaspoon olive oil, divided

1 rack of lamb (about 3 pounds), exterior fat trimmed

¼ cup chopped fresh apricots

¼ cup seedless grapes

¼ cup blueberries

2 tablespoons sesame seeds, toasted

¼ cup sliced fresh mint leaves

Juice of 2 lemons

1. Preheat the oven to 450°F.

2. In a small bowl, combine the cinnamon, black pepper, cumin, turmeric, ¼ teaspoon kosher salt, and the cloves.

3. Stir in 1 teaspoon olive oil. Smear the spice mixture all over the lamb.

4. Heat the remaining 1 tablespoon olive oil in a large, oven-safe, nonstick sauté pan over medium-high heat. Sear the lamb, fat-side down, until it is browned, 3 to 5 minutes.

5. Turn the lamb rack over so it's fat side up, and transfer the sauté pan to the oven. Roast the lamb until an instant-read thermometer inserted into the center reaches 145°F for medium-rare, 6 to 12 minutes.

6. Transfer the lamb to a cutting board, and let it rest for 10 minutes before cutting it into chops.

7. Meanwhile, in a small bowl, combine the apricots, grapes, blueberries, sesame seeds, and mint. Sprinkle with the lemon juice and the remaining ¼ teaspoon salt, and toss.

8. Serve the relish with the lamb chops.

REPAIR

Dinner

Sweet Potato Shepherd's Pie

SERVES 4 / PREP TIME: 20 MINUTES / COOK TIME: 25 MINUTES

This traditional Irish dish is usually topped with whipped white potatoes. Sweet potatoes make this Paleo-friendly and add a delicious, earthy sweetness to the dish.

3 large sweet potatoes, peeled and cut into ½-inch cubes

¼ cup unsweetened coconut milk

1 teaspoon sea salt, divided

½ teaspoon freshly ground black pepper, divided

2 tablespoons olive oil

1 onion, chopped

1 carrot, peeled and diced

1 pound ground lamb

1 garlic clove, minced

1 tablespoon tomato paste

½ teaspoon chopped fresh rosemary

¾ cup low-sodium chicken broth

Nut-free

REPAIR

Dinner

PER SERVING
CALORIES: 557
CARBS: 58G
FAT: 19G
PROTEIN: 37G
SUGAR: 4G

1. In a large pot, cover the sweet potatoes with water, and bring them to a boil over high heat. Boil until the potatoes are soft, about 15 minutes.

2. Drain the potatoes in a colander, and return them to the pot. Add the coconut milk, ½ teaspoon salt, and ¼ teaspoon black pepper.

3. Using a potato masher, mash the potatoes until smooth. Set aside.

4. Preheat the oven to 350°F.

5. In a large, ovenproof skillet, heat the olive oil over medium-high heat until it shimmers.

6. Add the onion and carrot and cook, stirring occasionally, until the vegetables are soft, about 5 minutes.

7. Add the lamb and cook, crumbling it with a spoon, until it is browned, about 5 minutes.

8. Add the garlic and cook, stirring constantly, until it is fragrant, about 30 seconds.

9. Add the tomato paste and cook, stirring constantly, until it begins to brown, another 2 minutes.

10. Add the rosemary and broth, scraping any browned bits from the bottom of the pan with a spoon. Season with the remaining ½ teaspoon salt and ¼ teaspoon pepper.

11. Simmer, stirring frequently, to blend the flavors, about 5 minutes.

12. Remove the pan from the heat. Gently spread the mashed sweet potatoes over the top of the ground lamb mixture in the sauté pan.

13. Bake for 25 minutes.

REPAIR

Dinner

Orange Beef Stir-Fry

SERVES 4 / PREP TIME: 20 MINUTES / COOK TIME: 5 MINUTES

This dish is quite spicy. Prepare the Do-It-Yourself Sriracha recipe (page 37) in advance, or look for sugar-free sriracha sauce at your local grocery store.

3 navel oranges

3 tablespoons gluten-free soy sauce

1 tablespoon arrowroot powder

1 teaspoon honey

3 tablespoons olive oil, divided

1 pound beef sirloin, trimmed and sliced against the grain into ⅛-inch-thick slices

4 garlic cloves, minced

2 tablespoons minced fresh ginger

1 teaspoon Do-It-Yourself Sriracha

6 scallions, thinly sliced

¼ cup sesame seeds

Nut-free

REPAIR

Dinner

PER SERVING
CALORIES: 468
CARBS: 27G
FAT: 23G
PROTEIN: 40G
SUGAR: 15G

1. With a small knife or vegetable peeler, carefully pare wide strips of zest from one of the oranges. Cut the zest into 1-inch strips, and set aside. Peel and cut the orange into rounds. Peel the remaining oranges, and cut them into rounds and set aside.

2. In a small bowl, combine the soy sauce, arrowroot powder, and honey and set aside.

3. In a large sauté pan or wok, heat 1 tablespoon olive oil over high heat until it shimmers. Add the beef and stir-fry just until it is no longer pink on the outside, about 1 minute. Transfer the beef to a plate and set aside.

4. Add the remaining 2 tablespoons oil to the pan. Add the garlic, ginger, sriracha, and the reserved orange zest. Stir-fry until fragrant, about 30 seconds.

5. Add the orange slices to the pan and stir. Add the soy sauce mixture and bring to a boil, stirring.

6. Add the scallions. Return the beef to the pan and toss to coat.

7. Serve sprinkled with sesame seeds.

Cowboy Steak with Grilled Peaches

SERVES 4 / PREP TIME: 10 MINUTES, PLUS 1 TO 8 HOURS TO MARINATE /
COOK TIME: 10 MINUTES

Flank steak takes very little cooking time to get to medium-rare. It just needs a quick sear in a cast iron pan. Use decaffeinated coffee in the recipe as well as gluten-free soy sauce to add deep flavor to the steak.

Technique tip: *Because it has very little fat marbling, flank steak can be a bit tough. To make the steak tender, don't overcook it. Then slice it against the grain. You can judge the grain of the meat by looking at how the meat fibers run up and down the steak. Slice crosswise to the long fibers to make them short and tender.*

3 tablespoons brewed decaffeinated coffee

2 tablespoons olive oil, divided

1 tablespoon gluten-free soy sauce

2 garlic cloves, minced

1½ teaspoons freshly ground black pepper

½ teaspoon liquid smoke

1 pound flank steak

4 medium peaches, halved and pitted

Nut-free

REPAIR

Dinner

PER SERVING
CALORIES: 322
CARBS: 10G
FAT: 17G
PROTEIN: 33G
SUGAR: 8G

1. In a deep-dish pie plate, whisk together the coffee, 1 tablespoon olive oil, soy sauce, garlic, pepper, and liquid smoke. Add the steak and turn to coat. Cover and refrigerate for at least 1 hour or up to 8 hours.

2. In a cast iron skillet, heat the remaining 1 tablespoon olive oil over medium-high heat until it shimmers.

3. Remove the steak, and discard the marinade. Cook the steak in the hot oil for 4 minutes per side for medium-rare. Transfer the steak to a cutting board, and let it rest for 10 minutes.

4. While the meat rests, put the peaches in the cast iron skillet, cut side down. Cook until they just begin to soften, about 1 minute. Carefully turn the peaches, and cook for 1 more minute.

5. Slice the steak across the grain, and serve with the peaches.

Cantaloupe Seed Drink

SERVES 4 / PREP TIME: 5 MINUTES

This refreshing drink is popular in Mexico. It uses both the flesh and seeds of the fruit. You can also make the drink with honeydew, casaba, or a similar melon for a nice variation. Garnish with a sprig of mint.

1 (2-pound) cantaloupe

3 cups cold water

Juice of 2 limes

1 tablespoon honey

Pinch of fine sea salt

Nut-free
Paleo-friendly
Vegetarian

REPAIR

Dessert

PER SERVING
CALORIES: 93
CARBS: 23G
FAT: 0G
PROTEIN: 2G
SUGAR: 22G

1. Scoop the melon flesh and seeds into a blender.

2. Add the water, lime juice, honey, and salt.

3. Blend until smooth.

4. Taste and add more lime juice if needed.

Chocolate-Banana Shake

SERVES 2 / PREP TIME: 5 MINUTES

This shake has bananas, which are high in carbohydrates and give you a quick hit of energy. Peel and slice the banana, and freeze it in a plastic container. Freezing it in slices makes it much easier for the blender to process the frozen banana. The banana will discolor in the freezer, but it will still taste fine and the cocoa powder will hide the discoloration.

2 cups frozen banana slices

¼ cup almond milk

2 tablespoons unsweetened cocoa powder

½ teaspoon vanilla extract

½ packet stevia

1. In a food processor or blender, combine the banana, almond milk, cocoa powder, vanilla, and stevia.

2. Process until smooth, about 30 to 60 seconds.

3. Serve immediately.

Vegan

REPAIR

Dessert

PER SERVING
CALORIES: 181
CARBS: 45G
FAT: 1G
PROTEIN: 3G
SUGAR: 31G

Orange Creamsicle Shake

SERVES 2 / PREP TIME: 10 MINUTES

The orange and vanilla flavors in this creamy shake will bring you back to when you were a kid eating a delicious Creamsicle. Although the recipe calls for coconut milk, if you prefer you can replace it with a different nondairy, non-soy, unsweetened milk, such as rice milk or almond milk.

2 cups crushed ice

1 cup unsweetened coconut milk

1 cup freshly squeezed orange juice

Zest of ½ orange

½ teaspoon vanilla extract

½ packet stevia

1. Put the crushed ice in a blender.
2. Add the coconut milk, orange juice, orange zest, vanilla, and stevia.
3. Blend on high until smooth, about 1 minute.

Nut-free
Vegan

REPAIR

Dessert

PER SERVING
CALORIES: 117
CARBS: 26G
FAT: 1G
PROTEIN: 9G
SUGAR: 29G

Kiwi-Strawberry Ice Pops

SERVES 8 / PREP TIME: 15 MINUTES, PLUS FREEZING TIME / COOK TIME: 5 MINUTES

While ice pops molds are helpful, you don't need them to make these delicious fruity pops. Instead, you can use paper cups, foil, and wooden sticks. Pour the purée into the paper cups, and cover them with foil. Then poke the sticks through the foil and freeze. When you're ready to eat the ice pops, remove the foil and peel away the paper cups.

1 cup water

¼ teaspoon powdered stevia

1 teaspoon grated fresh ginger

Juice of 1 lime

10 strawberries

2 kiwis, peeled and very thinly sliced

Nut-free
Paleo-friendly
Vegan

REPAIR

Dessert

PER SERVING
CALORIES: 17
CARBS: 4G
FAT: 0G
PROTEIN: 0G
SUGAR: 3G

1. In a small saucepan, combine the water, stevia, and ginger. Stir over high heat until the stevia dissolves and the mixture just simmers.

2. Remove from the heat, and let the mixture cool. Stir in the lime juice.

3. Line 8 individual frozen-treat molds or small (2-ounce) paper cups with slices of strawberry and kiwi. Fill each mold or cup with the lime mixture. Cover the mixture with foil, and insert the sticks.

4. Freeze until hard, and serve.

Honeydew and Berries

SERVES 4 / PREP TIME: 10 MINUTES

Honeydew melon and mint are a classic combination. Melon also tastes delicious with chopped fresh rosemary, which adds a different flavor profile to a simple fruit salad. You can substitute any type of melon you'd like in this salad.

1 honeydew melon, peeled, seeded, and cut into 1-inch pieces

Juice of 1 lemon

1 pint blueberries

½ cup chopped fresh mint

Nut-free
Paleo-friendly
Vegan

REPAIR

Dessert

PER SERVING
CALORIES: 178
CARBS: 45G
FAT: 1G
PROTEIN: 3G
SUGAR: 36G

1. In a medium bowl, toss the honeydew chunks with the lemon juice.
2. Gently stir in the blueberries and mint.

Fruit Medley

SERVES 4 / PREP TIME: 15 MINUTES

Combining fruit with vinegar balances the sweetness of the fruit. Balsamic vinegar pairs especially well with strawberries. Try an aged balsamic vinegar, which tends to be slightly sweeter and more concentrated than an unaged one. You can also use white balsamic vinegar.

Substitution tip: *Other fruits that work well with balsamic vinegar include peaches, nectarines, raspberries, blueberries, and blackberries. Feel free to substitute any of these fruits.*

Pinch of powdered stevia

2 tablespoons balsamic vinegar

1 pound fresh strawberries, hulled and sliced

2 bananas, peeled and sliced

3 medium kiwis, peeled and sliced

1. In a medium bowl, whisk the stevia into the vinegar.
2. Add the fruit and toss to coat.

Nut-free
Paleo-friendly
Vegan

REPAIR

Dessert

PER SERVING
CALORIES: 125
CARBS: 31G
FAT: 1G
PROTEIN: 2G
SUGAR: 18G

Blackberry-Pomegranate Salad

SERVES 2 / PREP TIME: 10 MINUTES, PLUS 2 HOURS TO MARINATE

Both blackberries and pomegranate seeds are loaded with beneficial antioxidants and phytonutrients. Blackberries are also high in vitamin C, while pomegranate seeds are high in dietary fiber, vitamin B₆, and vitamin C. Use fresh blackberries for this salad. Frozen berries are too watery and won't hold up well in a fresh fruit salad.

Technique tip: *To remove pomegranate seeds, split the pomegranate in half. Then hold the pomegranate, seed side down, over a bowl, and tap on the shell firmly with a wooden spoon, hitting it from multiple angles to extract all of the seeds. Many stores also sell the seeds already extracted from the shell.*

Nut-free
Paleo-friendly
Vegan

REPAIR

Dessert

PER SERVING
CALORIES: 124
CARBS: 29G
FAT: 0G
PROTEIN: 2G
SUGAR: 18G

1 cup fresh blackberries
1 cup fresh pomegranate seeds
Juice and finely grated zest of 1 orange

1. In a medium bowl, mix together the blackberries, pomegranate seeds, orange juice, and orange zest.
2. Allow to sit, covered, in the refrigerator for about 2 hours so the flavors combine.
3. Serve chilled.

Tea-Steeped Plums

SERVES 4 / PREP TIME: 15 MINUTES / COOK TIME: 5 MINUTES

Steeping plums in orange pekoe gives them a delicious scent of tea. If you prefer, you can try other decaffeinated or herbal teas, such as chamomile, cinnamon, or fruit-flavored tea. If you'd like this dessert a little sweeter, feel free to add a pinch of powdered stevia to the tea.

Ingredient tip: *When zesting oranges, avoid getting any of the white pith, which can be very bitter. Use a paring knife or a vegetable peeler with very light pressure to remove only the orange zest.*

1 navel orange

1 pound plums, halved and pitted

1 cup water

3 decaffeinated orange pekoe tea bags

1. Remove the zest from the orange in long strips. Peel and slice the orange into rounds.

2. Combine the orange zest, orange rounds, and plums in a medium saucepan. Add the water, and bring the mixture to a simmer. Remove the pan from the heat, and add the tea bags. Allow the mixture to steep for 3 minutes.

3. Remove the tea bags, and allow the plums to stand for a few more minutes. Remove the plums from the liquid with a slotted spoon and serve.

Nut-free
Paleo-friendly
Vegan

REPAIR

Dessert

PER SERVING
CALORIES: 56
CARBS: 14G
FAT: 0G
PROTEIN: 1G
SUGAR: 12G

Sautéed Apples with Ginger-Champagne Reduction

SERVES: 2 / PREP TIME: 5 MINUTES / COOK TIME: 15 MINUTES

Sautéing apples in a small amount of coconut oil allows the sugars to come to the surface, yielding a completely sweet flavor. While the apples caramelize, reduce champagne vinegar, a touch of pure maple syrup, and ground ginger in a small saucepan to serve drizzled over the apples for a delightfully sweet dessert.

2 tablespoons coconut oil

2 sweet-tart apples, stemmed, cored, and cut into thin slices lengthwise

1 cup champagne vinegar

1 tablespoon pure maple syrup

¼ teaspoon cinnamon

½ teaspoon ground ginger

Nut-free
Paleo-friendly
Vegan
Dairy-free

REPAIR

Dessert

PER SERVING
CALORIES: 187
CARBS: 34G
FAT: 5G
PROTEIN: 1G
SUGAR: 25G

1. In a medium-sized sauté pan, heat the coconut oil over medium-high heat until it shimmers, using a silicon pastry brush to spread the oil over the entire surface of the pan.

2. Add the apple slices to the hot pan and allow them to sit in contact with the pan without moving them until they are golden, about 5 minutes. Flip the apples and continue cooking them on the other side for another 2 to 3 minutes.

3. Meanwhile, in a small saucepan, whisk together the champagne vinegar, maple syrup, cinnamon, and ginger. Bring the mixture to a boil over medium-high heat, stirring frequently.

4. Continue cooking the vinegar mixture, stirring frequently, until it reduces to about a half cup, about 10 minutes.

5. Drizzle the warm vinegar mixture over the pears before serving.

Caramelized Pears with Spiced Balsamic Reduction

SERVES 2 / PREP TIME: 5 MINUTES / COOK TIME: 15 MINUTES

Caramelize Bosc or Anjou pears in a small amount of coconut oil. By leaving the pears in contact with the pan, the sugars come to the surface, yielding a complex sweet flavor. While the pears caramelize, reduce balsamic vinegar, a touch of honey, and ground spices in a small saucepan to serve drizzled over the pears for a delightfully sweet dessert.

2 teaspoons coconut oil

2 pears, stemmed, cored, and cut into thin slices lengthwise

1 cup balsamic vinegar

1 tablespoon raw organic honey

¼ teaspoon ground cinnamon

⅛ teaspoon freshly grated nutmeg

⅛ teaspoon ground ginger

Nut-free
Paleo-friendly
Vegan
Dairy-free

REPAIR

Dessert

PER SERVING
CALORIES: 218
CARBS: 42G
FAT: 5G
PROTEIN: 1G
SUGAR: 29G

1. In a medium-sized sauté pan, heat the coconut oil over medium-high heat until it shimmers, using a silicon pastry brush to spread the oil over the entire surface of the pan.

2. Add the pears to the hot pan and cook without moving them until they are golden, about 5 minutes. Flip the pears and continue cooking them on the other side for another 2 to 3 minutes.

3. Meanwhile, in a small saucepan, whisk together the balsamic vinegar, honey, cinnamon, nutmeg, and ginger. Bring the mixture to a boil over medium-high heat, stirring frequently.

4. Continue cooking the balsamic mixture, stirring frequently, until it reduces to about a half cup, about 10 minutes.

5. Drizzle the warm vinegar mixture over the pears before serving.

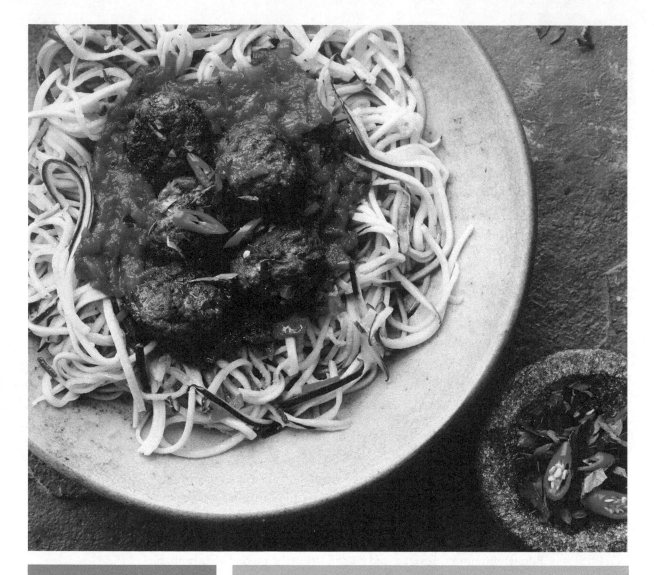

STAGE 2 RECIPES

Breakfast

Fresh Veggie Frittata 133
Summer Squash and Radish Hash with
   Poached Eggs 134
Poached Eggs Over Mushroom and
   Spinach Sauté 136
Breakfast Trout with Herbs and Eggs 138
Salmon Scramble 140
Canadian Bacon and Kale Pesto
   Roll-Ups 141
Turkey Breakfast Sausage 142
Sausage, Egg White, and Kale Breakfast
   Skillet 143
Spinach and Turkey Sausage Omelet 144
Baked Scotch Eggs with Spinach 146
Breakfast Bake with Turkey Sausage and
   Sweet Peppers 147
Turkey Bacon Cups with Egg White,
   Zucchini, and Mushroom Scramble 149
Breakfast Tacos 151

Lunch

Warm Asparagus and Ham Salad with
   Walnut Vinaigrette 152
Shrimp Cakes with Garlic Broccolini 153
Spicy Tuna Salad Lettuce Wraps 154
Gingered Chicken Salad 155
Spinach Salad with Chicken and Pesto
   Vinaigrette 157
Turkey Taco Salad 158

Slow Cooker Red Pepper Stuffed with
   Italian Seasoned Ground Turkey and
   Cauliflower 160
Chicken Fajitas 162
Slow Cooker Chicken Thighs with
   Cauliflower and Carrot Salad 164
Ground Beef and Cabbage Soup 165
Meatballs with Spinach 166
Roast Beef Roll-Ups 167

Snacks

Jicama Sticks with Chili and Lime 168
Zucchini Chips 169
Garlic Kale Chips 170
Daikon Radish Fries 171
Cauliflower "Popcorn" 172
Hardboiled Egg Whites with Garlicky
   Squash Purée 173
Spicy Pumpkin Seeds 175
Lemony Tuna and Radishes 176
Salmon Cucumber Rounds 177
Smoked Trout Wraps 178
Quick Pickled Cucumber and Turkey
   Roll-Ups 179
Ham, Basil, and Spinach Rolls 180

Dinner

Egg Drop Soup 181
Leafy Greens Soup 182
Vegetable Soup with Clams
   and Greens 183 »

STAGE 2 RECIPES *CONTINUED*

Fresh Veggie Frittata

SERVES 2 / PREP TIME: 5 MINUTES / COOK TIME: 15 MINUTES

While this recipe calls for spinach, zucchini, and red bell pepper, you can substitute whatever fresh, seasonal vegetables you have available. Be sure to add a leafy green, such as kale, to keep the level of antioxidants high.

7 egg whites

1 teaspoon unsweetened, unflavored almond milk

1 teaspoon olive oil

1 medium zucchini, cut into ¼-inch dice

¼ small red bell pepper, seeded and cut into ¼-inch dice

1 cup fresh baby spinach leaves

Fine sea salt

Freshly ground black pepper

1. Preheat the broiler. Place an oven rack in the middle of the oven.

2. In a small bowl, whisk together the egg whites and almond milk. Set aside.

3. In a medium ovenproof skillet, heat the olive oil over medium-high heat until it shimmers.

4. Add the zucchini and red bell pepper. Cook, stirring occasionally, until the vegetables are soft, about 5 minutes. Stir in the spinach, and cook until it wilts, about 1 minute longer.

5. Carefully pour the egg mixture over the top of the vegetables. Cook without stirring until the bottom half of the eggs sets, about 3 to 5 minutes.

6. Transfer the pan to the oven. Allow it to sit under the broiler until the top puffs and sets, about 3 more minutes.

7. Season with salt and pepper.

Nut-free
Paleo-friendly
Vegetarian

RELEASE

Breakfast

PER SERVING
CALORIES: 99
CARBS: 5G
FAT: 3G
PROTEIN: 14G
SUGAR: 3G

Summer Squash and Radish Hash with Poached Eggs

SERVES 2 / PREP TIME: 10 MINUTES / COOK TIME: 10 MINUTES

You can use any type of white-fleshed summer squash with this recipe, such as zucchini, patty pan squash, or yellow squash. While the squash cooks, poach the eggs so that the two are ready at the same time. Then serve the egg on top of the hash, and let the soft yolk run down over the hash to make a "sauce."

Technique tip: *To poach eggs, crack each egg into its own custard cup and set it aside while you get the water simmering. Bring water and about a tablespoon of vinegar to a simmer in a medium pot. When the water simmers, use a wooden spoon to begin swirling the water, making a whirlpool in the pot. As you swirl the water, hold the custard cup with the egg very close to the center of the vortex and slip it into the water. Repeat with each egg.*

Nut-free
Paleo-friendly
Vegetarian

RELEASE

Breakfast

PER SERVING
CALORIES: 246
CARBS: 13G
FAT: 19G
PROTEIN: 8G
SUGAR: 10G

2 tablespoons extra-virgin olive oil

1 pound summer squash, cut into ¼-inch cubes

2 large radishes, cut into ¼-inch cubes

½ sweet onion, diced

2 tablespoons vinegar

2 eggs

Sea salt

Freshly ground black pepper

2 tablespoons chopped fresh tarragon

1. Heat the olive oil in a large sauté pan over medium-high heat until it shimmers.

2. Add the squash, radishes, and onion, and cook, stirring occasionally, until the vegetables begin to brown, 8 to 10 minutes.

3. While the squash cooks, bring to a simmer a medium pot of water with 2 tablespoons of vinegar added.

4. Using the technique described in the tip for this recipe, poach the eggs for about 4 minutes, until the whites set.

5. Divide the summer squash between two plates.

6. Gently lift the poached eggs one at a time out of the water with a slotted spoon, and place them on top of the squash hash.

7. Season with salt and pepper.

8. Garnish with the chopped tarragon.

Poached Eggs Over Mushroom and Spinach Sauté

SERVES 2 / PREP TIME: 15 MINUTES / COOK TIME: 10 MINUTES

Sautéed mushrooms and spinach serve as a bed for a beautifully poached egg. (For instructions on poaching an egg, see Summer Squash and Radish Hash with Poached Eggs, page 134.) Use any type of mushrooms you wish. Favorites include button mushrooms, shiitakes, crimini, and chanterelles. To save time, buy baby spinach, which needs less cleaning and doesn't require you to remove the woody stems.

Nut-free
Paleo-friendly
Vegetarian

RELEASE

Breakfast

PER SERVING
CALORIES: 221
CARBS: 7G
FAT: 18G
PROTEIN: 10G
SUGAR: 2G

Ingredient tip: *For best results with mushrooms, leave them in contact with the pan without stirring them, until their liquids evaporate and they begin to brown, 7 to 10 minutes. Then continue cooking, stirring occasionally, until they are cooked through.*

2 tablespoons extra-virgin olive oil

2 cups sliced mushrooms

4 cups baby spinach

2 garlic cloves, minced

Juice of 1 lemon

Dash of red pepper flakes

Sea salt

Freshly ground black pepper

2 tablespoons vinegar

2 eggs

1. In a large sauté pan, heat the olive oil over medium-high heat until it shimmers. Add the mushrooms and cook, stirring occasionally, until they are browned, 7 to 10 minutes.

2. Add the spinach and cook, stirring frequently, until it begins to wilt, about 3 minutes.

3. Add the garlic and cook, stirring constantly, until it is fragrant, about 30 seconds.

4. Add the lemon juice and red pepper flakes, as well as salt and pepper. Cook, stirring constantly, for another 2 minutes.

5. Cover the sauté pan and set it aside.

6. In a large pot, bring water and the vinegar to a simmer over medium heat. Add the eggs and poach them for 4 minutes, until the whites have solidified.

7. Divide the spinach and mushrooms between two plates.

8. Using a slotted spoon, carefully lift the eggs out of the poaching liquid one at a time and place them on top of the spinach and mushroom mixture.

9. Season with more salt and pepper.

Breakfast Trout with Herbs and Eggs

SERVES 4 / PREP TIME: 15 MINUTES / COOK TIME: 10 MINUTES

When heated, a well-seasoned cast iron skillet requires almost no fat for cooking. Just a spray of olive oil will be enough for quick-cooking trout. Trout is a popular breakfast choice in many countries around the world. In this recipe, the trout pairs with flavorful fresh herbs that give it vibrant flavor and a pretty color. Be careful to remove the trout's pin bones (bones deep in the fillet that anchor the muscles) before cooking.

Technique tip: *Slightly older eggs peel more easily than fresh eggs when they are hardboiled. Use eggs that are at least 1 week old. To hard-boil eggs, place them in a single layer in the bottom of a pot and totally submerge them in water. Put the pot on the stove over medium-high heat. Bring the water to a boil. When the water boils, turn off the burner and cover the pot. Allow the eggs to sit in the hot water for 14 minutes. Then plunge the eggs into cold water to stop them from cooking further.*

Nut-free

RELEASE

Breakfast

PER SERVING
CALORIES: 279
CARBS: 1G
FAT: 17G
PROTEIN: 29G
SUGAR: 1G

¼ cup minced fresh flat-leaf parsley

¼ cup minced fresh basil

2 tablespoons minced fresh chives

2 tablespoons olive oil, divided

Juice of 1 lemon

¼ teaspoon ground white pepper

1 pound whole fresh trout, butterflied

½ cup low-sodium vegetable broth

4 hardboiled eggs, peeled and quartered

1. In a small bowl, combine the parsley, basil, chives, 1 tablespoon olive oil, the lemon juice, and the white pepper.

2. Lay the trout open on a work surface, skin side down, and spoon in the herb mixture in an even layer. Close the trout so its skin is facing out.

3. Heat a large cast iron skillet over medium-high heat. After a few minutes, add the remaining 1 tablespoon olive oil and allow it to heat to smoking hot.

4. Add the fish and cook until the one side is seared, 3 to 4 minutes. Turn the fish over and cook the other side until it is seared, 3 to 4 more minutes.

5. Remove the trout from the pan, and set it aside, tented with foil. Add the broth, and scrape up any browned bits from the bottom of the pan. Allow the broth to simmer until it is reduced to ¼ cup.

6. Divide the trout among 4 plates. Surround the trout with quartered hardboiled eggs. Spoon one-quarter of the broth over each piece of trout and serve.

RELEASE

Breakfast

Salmon Scramble

SERVES 1 / PREP TIME: 5 MINUTES / COOK TIME: 7 MINUTES

Many cultures around the world eat fish for breakfast. It is a terrific source of protein. Salmon is a great source of unsaturated fats and is high in omega-3 fatty acids and vitamin D. Find a smoked salmon that isn't cured with sugar in the brine.

Ingredient tip: *Cured fish keeps well in the refrigerator for about a week. Buy a large package of smoked salmon, take as much as you need for the recipe, and then wrap the rest tightly in plastic wrap for later use.*

Nut-free
Paleo-friendly

RELEASE

Breakfast

PER SERVING
CALORIES: 209
CARBS: 6G
FAT: 16G
PROTEIN: 14G
SUGAR: 2G

1 tablespoon olive oil

1 tablespoon finely chopped red onion

2 egg whites, beaten

1 tablespoon finely chopped fresh dill

½ teaspoon capers, rinsed and chopped

1 ounce smoked salmon

½ beefsteak tomato, chopped

1. In a small nonstick skillet, heat the olive oil over medium-high heat until it shimmers. Add the onion and cook, stirring, until it softens, about 3 minutes.

2. Add the egg whites, dill, and capers. Cook, stirring occasionally, until the whites are set, about 2 minutes. Stir in the salmon, and cook until it is heated through, another 1 to 2 minutes.

3. Serve the eggs topped with chopped tomato.

Canadian Bacon and Kale Pesto Roll-Ups

SERVES 4 / PREP TIME: 10 MINUTES

Make the pesto ahead of time for this dish, and store it, tightly sealed, in a container in the refrigerator for three to five days. Then spread the pesto on thinly sliced Canadian bacon for a quick, high-protein breakfast on the go.

2 cups kale, washed and stems removed

¼ cup fresh basil leaves

3 garlic cloves

¼ cup walnuts

1 tablespoons extra-virgin olive oil

Zest of 1 lemon

12 thin slices of lean Canadian bacon

Paleo-friendly

RELEASE

Breakfast

PER SERVING
CALORIES: 233
CARBS: 7G
FAT: 14G
PROTEIN: 20G
SUGAR: 1G

1. In a blender or a food processor fitted with a steel chopping blade, combine the kale, basil, garlic, walnuts, olive oil, and lemon zest.

2. Process on high speed until it forms a thin paste, about 1 minute.

3. Spread the pesto on Canadian bacon slices, and roll up the bacon around the pesto.

4. Serve 3 roll-ups per person.

Turkey Breakfast Sausage

SERVES 4 / PREP TIME: 10 MINUTES / COOK TIME: 20 MINUTES

Many brands of premade breakfast sausage contain brown sugar. Making your own is quick, easy, and flavorful, without any added sugar or preservatives. You can adjust the seasonings to suit your own tastes. Because the turkey sausage is very lean, you will need a little oil or nonstick cooking spray to cook it.

Ingredient tip: *For an even more flavorful sausage, replace the dried sage and marjoram with fresh sage and marjoram. If you are using fresh herbs, double the amount called for in the recipe—so add 2 teaspoons of fresh sage and 1 teaspoon of fresh marjoram.*

Nut-free
Paleo-friendly

RELEASE

Breakfast

PER SERVING
CALORIES: 253
CARBS: 0G
FAT: 16G
PROTEIN: 31G
SUGAR: 0G

1 pound ground turkey

1 teaspoon dried sage

½ teaspoon freshly ground black pepper

½ teaspoon dried marjoram

⅛ teaspoon ground nutmeg

⅛ teaspoon red pepper flakes

1 tablespoon olive oil

1. In a large bowl, combine the turkey, sage, black pepper, marjoram, nutmeg, and red pepper flakes.

2. Use your hands to carefully mix the herbs into the meat until the sausage is just combined. Do not overmix, or the sausage patties will be tough.

3. Form the sausage into 4 patties.

4. In a nonstick sauté pan, heat the olive oil over medium-high heat until it shimmers. Add the sausage patties to the pan. Cook without moving them, until the bottoms are browned, about 8 minutes.

5. Flip the sausages and cook them on the other side, without moving them, until they are cooked through, about 8 minutes.

Sausage, Egg White, and Kale Breakfast Skillet

SERVES 2 / PREP TIME: 10 MINUTES / COOK TIME: 15 MINUTES

This quick breakfast skillet dish has plenty of protein and the greens you need to get going. You can substitute low-fat store-bought sausage, but make sure it does not contain gluten or sugar.

Substitution tip: *You can replace the kale with any dark leafy green, such as Swiss chard or spinach.*

2 tablespoons olive oil, divided
½ pound uncooked Turkey Breakfast Sausage (page 142)
½ onion, chopped
2 cups kale, stems removed and leaves chopped
2 garlic cloves, minced
6 egg whites, beaten
Fine sea salt
Freshly ground black pepper

Nut-free
Paleo-friendly

RELEASE

Breakfast

PER SERVING
CALORIES: 209
CARBS: 8G
FAT: 15G
PROTEIN: 13G
SUGAR: 2G

1. In a large nonstick skillet, heat 1 tablespoon olive oil over medium-high heat until it shimmers. Add the turkey sausage and cook, crumbling with a spoon, until it is browned, about 5 minutes.

2. Remove the sausage from the pan, and set it aside. Add the remaining 1 tablespoon olive oil, and heat until it shimmers.

3. Add the onion and kale, and cook until the vegetables soften, about 5 minutes.

4. Add the garlic and cook, stirring constantly, until it is fragrant, about 30 seconds. Reduce the heat to medium.

5. Return the sausage to the pan, and add the egg whites. Cook, stirring frequently, until the eggs are set, about 3 more minutes.

6. Season with salt and pepper.

Spinach and Turkey Sausage Omelet

SERVES 4 / PREP TIME: 10 MINUTES / COOK TIME: 15 MINUTES

Use the Turkey Breakfast Sausage recipe to make this quick and easy omelet. Sauté the turkey sausage and spinach mixture first, and set it aside. Then use the same pan to cook the eggs. For best results, use a nonstick pan to make omelets.

2 tablespoons olive oil, divided

¼ pound uncooked Turkey Breakfast Sausage (page 142)

2 cups baby spinach

2 garlic cloves, minced

4 eggs

4 egg whites

¼ teaspoon sea salt

¼ teaspoon freshly ground pepper

Nut-free
Paleo-friendly

RELEASE

Breakfast

PER SERVING
CALORIES: 147
CARBS: 2G
FAT: 12G
PROTEIN: 10G
SUGAR: 1G

1. In a large, nonstick sauté pan, heat 1 tablespoon olive oil over medium-high heat until it shimmers.

2. Add the turkey sausage and cook, crumbling with a spoon, until it browns, 5 to 7 minutes.

3. Add the spinach and cook, stirring occasionally, until it wilts, about 2 minutes.

4. Add the garlic and cook, stirring constantly, until it is fragrant, about 30 seconds.

5. Using a slotted spoon, remove the sausage and spinach mixture from the pan, and set it aside on a platter.

6. Return the pan to the burner, and reduce the heat to medium. Add the remaining 1 tablespoon olive oil to the pan, and let it warm up.

7. Meanwhile, in a medium bowl, whisk together the eggs, egg whites, salt, and pepper.

8. Pour the egg mixture in the hot pan, and let it cook, without touching or stirring, until the egg begins to set around the edges. Then very carefully pull back the edges of the eggs with a spatula, allow the runny eggs from the center of the pan to fill the gaps, and continue cooking until the eggs are solid across the entire surface.

9. Add the sausage mixture on top, along one side of the eggs in the pan. Flip the other side of the eggs over the top of the filling, using a spatula.

10. Cut into slices and serve.

Baked Scotch Eggs with Spinach

SERVES 4 / PREP TIME: 10 MINUTES / COOK TIME: 30 MINUTES

Scotch eggs are a popular meal or appetizer in British gastropubs. Traditionally, a Scotch egg is a hardboiled egg wrapped in sausage, dipped in crushed cornflakes or breadcrumbs, and deep-fried. This low-carb version is baked rather than fried, and adds healthy spinach and herbs to the sausage.

Serving tip: *In pubs, Scotch eggs are served with mustard for dipping. Choose a hearty, grainy mustard for big flavor.*

1 cup frozen spinach, thawed and drained

1 pound uncooked Turkey Breakfast Sausage (page 142)

1 tablespoon chopped fresh thyme

1 tablespoon chopped fresh rosemary

4 hardboiled eggs, peeled

Nut-free
Paleo-friendly

RELEASE

Breakfast

PER SERVING
CALORIES: 291
CARBS: 2G
FAT: 17G
PROTEIN: 37G
SUGAR: 0G

1. Preheat the oven to 400°F.

2. Drain the spinach in a colander, pushing on it with a spoon to remove any excess water. Chop the spinach finely.

3. In a large bowl, combine the turkey sausage, spinach, thyme, and rosemary, using your hands to mix and incorporate the herbs and spinach into the sausage.

4. Divide the sausage into four equal parts. Form each into a thin patty. Wrap each patty around an egg until it covers the egg completely.

5. Bake the eggs on a rimmed baking sheet until the sausage is cooked through, 25 to 30 minutes.

Breakfast Bake with Turkey Sausage and Sweet Peppers

SERVES 8 / PREP TIME: 10 MINUTES / COOK TIME: 40 MINUTES

This casserole keeps well, so you can make extra. Cover and store it in your refrigerator for up to five days. That way, it's easy to eat breakfast on the run. Just reheat a serving of the casserole, and your day will be off to a healthy start.

Substitution tip: *While the recipe calls for sweet red bell peppers, you can use any type and color of sweet bell pepper you like. Mix them together for a lovely multicolor effect.*

6 eggs

6 egg whites

1 tablespoon Dijon mustard

½ teaspoon sea salt

¼ teaspoon freshly ground black pepper

1 teaspoon garlic powder

Dash of cayenne pepper

1 tablespoon olive oil

1 pound uncooked Turkey Breakfast Sausage (page 142)

1 sweet red bell pepper, seeded and chopped

½ onion, chopped

1 cup grated zucchini

Nut-free
Paleo-friendly

RELEASE

Breakfast

PER SERVING
CALORIES: 197
CARBS: 2G
FAT: 12G
PROTEIN: 23G
SUGAR: 2G

1. Preheat oven to 375°F. Line a 9-by-9-inch square baking dish with parchment paper.

2. In a large bowl, whisk together the eggs, egg whites, mustard, salt, pepper, garlic powder, and cayenne. Set aside.

3. In a large, nonstick sauté pan, heat the olive oil over medium-high heat until it shimmers. Add the breakfast sausage and cook, breaking it up with a spoon, until it browns, about 5 minutes. »

Breakfast Bake with Turkey Sausage and Sweet Peppers *continued*

4. Add the bell pepper and onion, and continue cooking, stirring occasionally, until the vegetables are soft, about 5 more minutes.

5. Gently stir the sausage and pepper mixture into the egg mixture. Stir in the zucchini.

6. Pour the mixture into the prepared baking pan. Bake until the center sets, about 30 minutes.

RELEASE

Breakfast

Turkey Bacon Cups with Egg White, Zucchini, and Mushroom Scramble

SERVES 2 / PREP TIME: 15 MINUTES / COOK TIME: 20 MINUTES

Form these nifty turkey bacon cups on the bottom side of a muffin tin that's covered with foil. Then you can fill the cups with any number of delicious breakfast foods. In this recipe, the filling is scrambled egg whites, mushroom, and zucchini.

Ingredient tip: *Choose a low-salt, thin-sliced turkey bacon for these bacon cups. Each cup uses three strips of bacon. Make several of the cups, and then refrigerate them, tightly sealed, for up to five days to use with other fillings.*

6 slices lean turkey bacon

4 egg whites

1 tablespoon Dijon mustard

1 tablespoon olive oil

½ cup chopped zucchini

½ cup chopped mushrooms

½ onion, chopped

Sea salt

Freshly ground black pepper

Nut-free
Paleo-friendly

RELEASE

Breakfast

PER SERVING
CALORIES: 177
CARBS: 4G
FAT: 9G
PROTEIN: 18G
SUGAR: 2G

1. Preheat the oven to 325°F.

2. Line the bottom of a standard-size muffin tin with aluminum foil. Place the muffin tin upside-down on a rimmed baking sheet.

3. Place one strip of bacon across the underside of one cup on the muffin tin. Place another piece of bacon across it to form a cross. Now, add a third strip of bacon next to the cross piece. Weave the bacon together to form a basket weave over the tin.

4. Repeat on a second cup. Each cup will have three strips of bacon.

5. Put the cookie sheet with the bacon-wrapped muffin tins in the oven and bake until the bacon is brown and crispy, about 10 minutes. »

Turkey Bacon Cups with Egg White, Zucchini, and Mushroom Scramble
continued

6. Remove from the oven, and allow to cool for about 10 minutes before unmolding the bacon cups.

7. Meanwhile, in a medium bowl, whisk together the egg whites and mustard, and set aside.

8. When the bacon cups are ready, in a large sauté pan, heat the olive oil over medium-high heat until it shimmers. Add the zucchini, mushrooms, and onion. Cook, stirring occasionally, until the vegetables soften and begin to brown, 5 to 7 minutes.

9. Add the eggs and cook, stirring constantly, until the eggs are set, 3 to 4 minutes.

10. Season with salt and pepper.

11. Spoon the eggs into the bacon cups to serve.

RELEASE

Breakfast

Breakfast Tacos

SERVES 2 / PREP TIME: 10 MINUTES / COOK TIME: 5 MINUTES

Lettuce leaves make a fine substitute for tortillas during the stages that call for limited carbohydrates. This breakfast comes together as quickly as a bowl of cereal, and it keeps you satisfied all morning.

Time-saving tip: *You can buy it premade in the produce section of the grocery store. Check the ingredients to make sure it is sugar-free.*

For the pico de gallo

½ red onion, finely minced

1 jalapeño pepper, seeded and finely minced

1 large tomato, seeded and diced

¼ cup chopped fresh cilantro

Juice of 1 lime

Fine sea salt

For the tacos

Nonstick cooking spray

4 egg whites, scrambled

2 romaine lettuce leaves

4 slices reduced-fat turkey bacon, cooked and chopped

2 tablespoons pico de gallo

½ avocado, sliced

Nut-free
Paleo-friendly

RELEASE

Breakfast

PER SERVING
CALORIES: 188
CARBS: 6G
FAT: 11G
PROTEIN: 14G
SUGAR: 2G

To make the pico de gallo

1. In a small bowl, combine the onion, jalapeño, tomato, cilantro, and lime juice.

2. Season with salt. Set aside.

To make the tacos

1. Heat a nonstick pan over medium heat. Lightly coat the pan with cooking spray.

2. Add the egg whites, and cook until they are opaque, about 2 minutes.

3. Divide the scrambled eggs among the lettuce leaves.

4. Top with bacon, pico de gallo, and avocado.

Warm Asparagus and Ham Salad with Walnut Vinaigrette

SERVES 4 / PREP TIME: 15 MINUTES / COOK TIME: 10 MINUTES

Use extra-lean ham or turkey ham for this salad, cut into thin slices. When paired with chopped walnuts and a vinaigrette with walnut oil, along with tender asparagus, this is a delicious and filling lunch. While the recipe calls for steaming the asparagus, you can also grill or roast it for a smoky flavor.

Paleo-friendly

RELEASE

Lunch

PER SERVING
CALORIES: 166
CARBS: 7G
FAT: 8G
PROTEIN: 16G
SUGAR: 2G

1 pound asparagus, woody ends removed, cut into 1-inch pieces
½ pound extra-lean ham, cubed
Juice of 1 lemon
½ cup red wine vinegar
2 garlic cloves, finely minced
1 tablespoon finely minced shallot
½ teaspoon sea salt
¼ teaspoon freshly ground black pepper
¼ cup walnut oil
2 tablespoons finely chopped walnuts

1. Place a steamer basket in a large pot with about 1 inch of water. Bring the water to a simmer over medium-high heat.

2. Add the asparagus to the steamer basket. Cover and steam until the asparagus is soft, 5 to 10 minutes depending on the thickness of the stalks.

3. While the asparagus steams, fill a large bowl with water and ice.

4. When the asparagus is done cooking, quickly plunge it into the ice water to stop the cooking, and drain it in a colander. Put the warm asparagus into a large bowl with the ham.

5. In a small bowl, whisk together the lemon juice, vinegar, garlic, shallot, salt, pepper, and walnut oil.

6. Pour the dressing over the asparagus and ham. Add the walnuts and toss to combine. Serve warm or cold.

Shrimp Cakes with Garlic Broccolini

SERVES 6 / PREP TIME: 15 MINUTES / COOK TIME: 15 MINUTES

Broccolini is a long, thin Asian broccoli that is tender and has a milder flavor than broccoli. It is available in the produce section of most grocery stores. If you can't find broccolini, you can use broccoli instead.

Time-saving tip: *These shrimp cakes pack easily for lunches away from home.*

1 pound uncooked shrimp, peeled and deveined

2 teaspoons grated fresh ginger

1 bunch fresh chives, coarsely chopped

Juice of 1 lime

1 teaspoon Do-It-Yourself Sriracha (page 37) or sugar-free sriracha sauce

1 egg, beaten

2 bunches broccolini (about 1 pound), trimmed and cut into 3-inch pieces

1 tablespoon olive oil

6 garlic cloves, sliced

1. In a food processor, pulse the shrimp, ginger, chives, lime juice, and sriracha until the mixture begins to come together, or chop the mixture very finely on a large cutting board.

2. Scrape the shrimp mixture into a bowl and stir in the egg. Form into 6 patties. Set aside.

3. Place a steamer basket in a large saucepan, and add water to a level just below the bottom of the steamer. Bring the water to a boil over high heat. Add the broccolini, cover, and cook 4 minutes. Remove the broccolini, and rinse with cold water to stop it from cooking.

4. In a large, nonstick sauté pan, heat the olive oil over medium-high heat until it shimmers. Add the broccolini and cook until it caramelizes, about 5 minutes. Add the garlic and cook until it is fragrant, about 30 seconds. Push the broccolini to the side of the pan.

5. Add the shrimp cakes in a single layer (you may need to do this in batches), and cook until they begin to brown, about 3 minutes. Turn the cakes over, and repeat on the other side.

6. Serve the shrimp cakes with the broccolini on the side.

Nut-free

RELEASE

Lunch

PER SERVING
CALORIES: 164
CARBS: 8G
FAT: 5G
PROTEIN: 21G
SUGAR: 2G

Spicy Tuna Salad Lettuce Wraps

SERVES 4 / PREP TIME: 10 MINUTES

Tuna is full of healthy omega-3s. To keep the fat content low, choose water-packed tuna. To keep this tuna salad low-carb, serve it wrapped in large romaine or butter lettuce leaves. Use the Easy Homemade Mayonnaise recipe (page 37), and you'll know it's sugar-free, as well. You can adjust the amount of heat in this tuna salad by adjusting the amount of sriracha. If you like it spicier, just add more than the recipe calls for.

2 tablespoons Easy Homemade Mayonnaise

¼ teaspoon Do-It-Yourself Sriracha (page 37) or sugar-free sriracha sauce

Juice and zest of 1 lemon

½ teaspoon sea salt

¼ teaspoon freshly ground black pepper

12 ounces canned water-packed tuna, drained and rinsed

2 stalks celery, finely chopped

3 scallions, finely chopped

2 medium radishes, finely chopped

4 to 8 large lettuce leaves

1. In a small bowl, whisk together the mayonnaise, sriracha, lemon juice and zest, salt, and pepper. Set aside.

2. In a large bowl, mix the tuna, celery, scallions, and radishes. Toss with the mayonnaise mixture to combine.

3. Wrap the tuna salad in large lettuce leaves to serve.

Nut-free

RELEASE

Lunch

PER SERVING
CALORIES: 116
CARBS: 4G
FAT: 5G
PROTEIN: 18G
SUGAR: 1G

Gingered Chicken Salad

SERVES 4 / PREP TIME: 15 MINUTES, PLUS 1 HOUR TO OVERNIGHT TO MARINATE /
COOK TIME: 20 MINUTES

Prep the chicken in the morning, and leave it to marinate, covered, in the refrigerator all day. If you prefer, you can also marinate the chicken for one hour before cooking, although longer marinating results in more intense flavors. Bring the chicken to room temperature before proceeding.

Substitution tip: *Any salad greens will work for this salad, such as spinach, butter lettuce, or arugula. Add them to the romaine, radicchio, and frisée, or swap them.*

2 tablespoons low-sodium vegetable broth

2 tablespoons minced fresh ginger

Zest of 2 oranges, divided

Zest of 1 lime, divided

1 pound chicken breast tenders

Fine sea salt

Freshly ground black pepper

1 tablespoon white wine vinegar

1 head romaine lettuce, cored and chopped

1 small head radicchio or chicory, cored and chopped

1 small head frisée lettuce, cored and chopped

Nut-free

RELEASE

Lunch

PER SERVING
CALORIES: 132
CARBS: 6G
FAT: 1G
PROTEIN: 24G
SUGAR: 2G

1. In a dish that has a cover, whisk together the broth, ginger, 1 tablespoon orange zest, and 1 teaspoon lime zest.

2. Season the chicken with salt and pepper, and add it to the broth marinade. Turn the chicken to coat, cover, and refrigerate it 1 hour or overnight.

3. Heat a cast iron skillet over medium-high heat. Remove the chicken from the marinade, scraping off as much of the marinade as you can. Discard the marinade.

4. Put the chicken in a single layer in the hot pan. Cook for 8 minutes. Turn the chicken, and cook until it is cooked through, about 8 minutes more. Remove the chicken from the pan, and let it rest for a few minutes before cutting into 1-inch pieces. »

Gingered Chicken Salad *continued*

5. Meanwhile, in a small bowl, whisk together the remaining 1 tablespoon orange zest and 1 teaspoon lime zest, and the vinegar. Season the vinaigrette with salt and pepper.

6. In a large bowl, combine the lettuce, radicchio, and frisée. Pour the vinaigrette over the top, and toss to coat. Add the chicken to the salad bowl, and toss again to combine.

RELEASE

Lunch

Spinach Salad with Chicken and Pesto Vinaigrette

SERVES 3 / PREP TIME: 20 MINUTES

Use deli rotisserie chicken for this salad, which makes it come together quickly. To take the salad to work, pack the vinaigrette and greens separately, and then give the dressing a shake to mix it up before you pour it on the salad. The addition of red peppers gives bright color to this tasty salad.

Substitution tip: *You can use any leafy green in place of the spinach. For example, try arugula or romaine lettuce, or a blend of both.*

4 cups baby spinach

2 cups cooked chicken, skin removed

1 red pepper, seeded and chopped

1 carrot, peeled and thinly sliced

1 cup loosely packed basil leaves

2 tablespoons pine nuts

4 garlic cloves

2 tablespoons olive oil

¼ teaspoon sea salt

¼ teaspoon freshly ground black pepper

¼ cup red wine vinegar

Paleo-friendly

RELEASE

Lunch

PER SERVING
CALORIES: 199
CARBS: 8G
FAT: 10G
PROTEIN: 20G
SUGAR: 2G

1. In a large bowl, combine the spinach, chicken, red pepper, and carrot. Toss to mix.

2. In a blender or the bowl of a food processor fitted with a metal chopping blade, process the basil, pine nuts, garlic, olive oil, salt, and pepper until it makes a thin paste.

3. Put the pesto in a small bowl, and add the red wine vinegar. Whisk to combine.

4. Pour the dressing over the salad, and toss to combine.

Turkey Taco Salad

SERVES 4 / PREP TIME: 20 MINUTES / COOK TIME: 10 MINUTES

Some taco seasoning mixes contain gluten and sugar, but it's really easy to make your own spice blend to season your ground turkey. Then pile the turkey high with taco salad fixings, including tomatoes, scallions, iceberg lettuce, and salsa. Finish with a squeeze of lime juice for a nice hit of acidity.

Time-saving tip: *If you don't feel like chopping a bunch of vegetables for the salad, you can substitute premade pico de gallo, which you can find in the produce section at your local grocery.*

Nut-free
Paleo-friendly

RELEASE

Lunch

PER SERVING
CALORIES: 226
CARBS: 7G
FAT: 12G
PROTEIN: 24G
SUGAR: 3G

For the turkey

1 tablespoon olive oil

1 pound lean ground turkey

1 tablespoon chili powder

¼ teaspoon garlic powder

Dash of cayenne pepper

½ teaspoon dried oregano

½ teaspoon ground cumin

¼ teaspoon onion powder

½ teaspoon sea salt

¼ teaspoon freshly ground black pepper

½ cup water

For the salad

4 cups shredded iceberg lettuce

1 large beefsteak tomato, chopped

4 scallions, chopped

4 tablespoons prepared salsa

1 lime, cut into 4 wedges

To make the turkey

1. In a large nonstick sauté pan, heat the olive oil over medium-high heat until it shimmers. Add the turkey and cook, crumbling with a spoon, until it is browned, about 6 minutes.

2. In a small bowl, combine the chili powder, garlic powder, cayenne, oregano, cumin, onion powder, salt, and pepper. Mix well.

3. Add the seasoning blend and the water to the turkey, and stir to combine well. Simmer for about 3 minutes, until the turkey is well-seasoned and the water has evaporated.

To make the salad

1. In a large bowl, combine the lettuce, tomato, and scallions. Toss to combine.

2. Add the ground turkey mixture to the lettuce, and toss to combine.

3. Serve each portion with a tablespoon of salsa and a wedge of lime.

RELEASE

Lunch

Slow Cooker Red Pepper Stuffed with Italian Ground Turkey and Cauliflower

SERVES 4 / PREP TIME: 15 MINUTES / COOK TIME: 4 TO 10 HOURS IN A SLOW COOKER

Rice is too high in carbs for this stage of the diet. Instead, cauliflower makes a nice base for these stuffed peppers. You will "rice" the cauliflower in a food processor to give it a rice-like texture and shape.

Substitution tip: *Substitute green peppers for the red if you prefer. The green peppers will be slightly less sweet, with a more vegetal flavor.*

1 head of cauliflower, broken into florets

2 tablespoons olive oil

1 pound lean ground turkey

½ onion, finely minced

4 garlic cloves, finely minced

2 tablespoons Italian seasoning, divided

Sea salt

Freshly ground black pepper

4 red bell peppers, tops removed, seeded

2 (14-ounce) cans sugar-free, gluten-free tomato sauce

Dash of red pepper flakes

1 teaspoon garlic powder

¼ cup chopped fresh basil

1. In a food processor fitted with a metal chopping blade, pulse the cauliflower florets for 10 one-second pulses, or until the cauliflower resembles rice in size. Set aside. If you don't have a food processor, use a chef's knife to chop the cauliflower into very small pieces about the size of grains of rice.

2. In a large, nonstick sauté pan, heat the olive oil over medium-high heat until it shimmers. Add the ground turkey and cook, breaking it up with the side of a spoon, until it browns, about 5 minutes.

3. Add the onion and cauliflower. Cook, stirring occasionally, until the onion is soft, about 5 minutes.

4. Add the garlic, 1 tablespoon Italian seasoning, and salt and pepper. Cook, stirring constantly, until the garlic is fragrant, about 30 seconds.

5. Fill the bell peppers with the ground turkey mixture. Put them in the bottom of a slow cooker.

6. In a medium bowl, whisk together the tomato sauce, red pepper flakes, garlic powder, and remaining 1 tablespoon Italian seasoning.

7. Carefully add the sauce to the slow cooker, pouring it around the peppers.

8. Cover the slow cooker, and cook on high for 4 to 5 hours or low for 8 to 10 hours.

9. Using tongs, remove the peppers from the sauce in the slow cooker. Stir the fresh basil into the sauce.

10. Serve the peppers with the sauce spooned over the top.

RELEASE

Lunch

Chicken Fajitas

SERVES 6 / PREP TIME: 15 MINUTES, PLUS 30 MINUTES TO 8 HOURS TO MARINATE /
COOK TIME: 50 MINUTES

*Worcestershire sauce adds great depth to the marinade in this recipe. If you don't
have any on hand, substitute gluten-free soy sauce. The marinade works equally
well with shrimp—although you should reduce the marinating time to 10 minutes.*

8 tablespoons low-sodium chicken broth, divided

Juice of 1 lime

2 tablespoons Worcestershire sauce

1 garlic clove, minced

¾ teaspoon fine sea salt, divided

½ teaspoon freshly ground black pepper

½ teaspoon ground cumin

½ teaspoon chili powder

2 pounds boneless, skinless chicken breasts

2 onions, cut into thin half moons

1 teaspoon dried thyme

1 yellow bell pepper, seeded and cut into ½-inch strips

1 red bell pepper, seeded and cut into ½-inch strips

1 green bell pepper, seeded and cut into ½-inch strips

¼ cup chopped fresh cilantro

1. In a small bowl, whisk together 4 tablespoons broth, lime juice,
   Worcestershire sauce, garlic, ½ teaspoon salt, pepper, cumin, and
   chili powder.

2. Put the chicken in a zip-top bag, and pour the marinade over the top.
   Seal the bag and turn to coat. Marinate the chicken in the refrigerator
   for at least 30 minutes or up to 8 hours.

3. In a large, nonstick sauté pan, heat 2 tablespoons broth over medium-
   high heat. Add the chicken and cook until it begins to brown, about
   10 minutes. Turn the chicken over. Reduce the heat to medium. Cover
   and continue cooking until the chicken is cooked through, about 10 more
   minutes. Remove the chicken from the pan with tongs, and set it aside on
   a platter, tented with foil.

4. Meanwhile, heat the remaining 2 tablespoons broth over medium-high heat in the same nonstick skillet. Add the onions, and cook until they begin to look translucent, about 6 minutes. Add the remaining $\frac{1}{4}$ teaspoon salt and the thyme. Cover, reduce the heat to low, and cook, stirring occasionally, for 10 minutes.

5. Remove the lid, return the heat to medium-high and add the bell peppers. Add additional broth, if needed, to prevent scorching. Cook, stirring occasionally, until the peppers begin to soften and caramelize, about 10 minutes.

6. Cut the chicken into thin slices, and sprinkle with cilantro. Serve with the peppers and onions.

Slow Cooker Chicken Thighs with Cauliflower and Carrot Salad

SERVES 4 / PREP TIME: 15 MINUTES / COOK TIME: 8 HOURS IN A SLOW COOKER

This recipe is reminiscent of an Indian curry. If you have cardamom and coriander on hand, add ½ teaspoon of each to the spice mix for more of a curry flavor. If you don't have a nonstick baking sheet, line a regular baking sheet with parchment paper.

Substitution tip: *You can use fresh ginger for this recipe, but jarred minced ginger makes this dinner come together in a flash.*

Nut-free
Paleo-friendly

RELEASE

Lunch

PER SERVING
CALORIES: 355
CARBS: 11G
FAT: 15G
PROTEIN: 43G
SUGAR: 5G

1 tablespoon olive oil

1 tablespoon mustard powder

1 teaspoon grated fresh ginger

½ teaspoon ground cumin

½ teaspoon ground cloves

½ teaspoon freshly ground black pepper

½ teaspoon cayenne pepper

4 boneless, skinless chicken thighs, cut into 1-inch pieces

1 head cauliflower, cored and cut into 1-inch pieces

4 medium carrots, peeled and cut on the diagonal into 1-inch pieces

1. In a small bowl, combine the olive oil, mustard powder, ginger, cumin, cloves, black pepper, and cayenne.

2. Put the chicken, cauliflower, and carrots in a slow cooker. Add the oil and spice mixture. Stir to combine.

3. Turn the slow cooker to low, and cook for 8 hours.

Ground Beef and Cabbage Soup

SERVES 6 / PREP TIME: 10 MINUTES / COOK TIME: 30 MINUTES

This hearty soup uses extra-lean ground beef, which is 10 percent fat or less. Check at your grocery store, and choose the lowest-fat ground beef available. Use Napa cabbage or green cabbage for the soup. Canned tomatoes work very well here, and they add delicious flavor. Feel free to add any nonstarchy vegetables you like to this recipe.

1 tablespoon olive oil

1 onion, chopped

1 pound extra-lean ground beef

3 garlic cloves, finely minced

1 (15-ounce) can crushed tomatoes, undrained

6 cups low-sodium chicken broth

2 carrots, peeled and sliced

1 celery stalk, sliced

2 cups finely chopped cabbage

1 teaspoon dried thyme

1 teaspoon sea salt

½ teaspoon freshly ground black pepper

Nut-free

RELEASE

Lunch

PER SERVING
CALORIES: 247
CARBS: 13G
FAT: 9G
PROTEIN: 27G
SUGAR: 8G

1. In a large soup pot, heat the olive oil over medium-high heat until it shimmers. Add the onion and cook, stirring occasionally, until it is soft, about 5 minutes.

2. Add the ground beef and cook, crumbling with the spoon, until it is browned, about 5 minutes.

3. Add the garlic and cook until it is fragrant, about 30 seconds.

4. Add the tomatoes and their juice, broth, carrots, celery, cabbage, thyme, salt, and pepper. Scrape up any browned bits from the bottom of the pan.

5. Cook, stirring occasionally, until the vegetables soften, about 15 minutes more.

Meatballs with Spinach

SERVES 8 / PREP TIME: 15 MINUTES / COOK TIME: 25 MINUTES

Any dark green, leafy vegetable can be added to the meatballs for extra nutrients and flavor. If your garden is brimming with fresh spinach, chard, or kale, remove the coarse stems and cut the greens into small pieces.

1 (16-ounce) package frozen spinach, thawed

1 egg

2 pounds extra-lean ground beef

½ onion, minced

4 garlic cloves, minced

½ packed cup chopped fresh basil

½ cup chopped fresh flat-leaf parsley

1 tablespoon dried oregano

1 teaspoon ground cumin

½ teaspoon fine sea salt

½ teaspoon freshly ground black pepper

⅓ cup low-sodium chicken broth

2 cups canned crushed tomatoes, drained

¼ teaspoon red pepper flakes

Sea salt

Freshly ground black pepper

Nut-free

RELEASE

Lunch

PER SERVING
CALORIES: 184
CARBS: 7G
FAT: 5G
PROTEIN: 26G
SUGAR: 2G

1. Drain and squeeze out as much moisture as possible from the spinach.

2. Whisk the egg in a large bowl. Add the drained spinach, ground beef, onion, garlic, basil, parsley, oregano, cumin, ½ teaspoon salt, and ½ teaspoon pepper. Using your hands, mix to combine.

3. Divide the meat into 16 portions, and roll each into a ball.

4. Heat a large, nonstick skillet over medium-high heat. Add the broth, and cook for 1 minute. Add the meatballs, leaving some space between each one, and cook, turning occasionally, until all the sides are evenly browned, 15 to 20 minutes.

5. Meanwhile, in a small saucepan, heat the tomatoes and red pepper flakes over low heat until warmed through. Season with salt and pepper.

6. Spoon the tomatoes over the meatballs, and serve.

Roast Beef Roll-Ups

SERVES 6 / PREP TIME: 10 MINUTES / COOK TIME: 5 MINUTES

In Germany, beef is stuffed with pickles. In Japan, it is served with asparagus. This recipe is easily adaptable to any vegetable that would be at home on a crudité plate. This is a great on-the-go snack or lunch, and can be made beforehand then refrigerated. Take the dressing in a separate container as a dipping sauce.

Ingredient tip: *Some deli roast beef contains wheat or gluten in the saline solution that keeps it moist and flavorful. Ask for gluten-free roast beef at the deli counter.*

16 asparagus spears, trimmed

16 slices deli roast beef

½ cup balsamic vinegar

2 tablespoons Dijon mustard

1. Place a steamer basket in a large saucepan, and add water to a level just below the bottom of the steamer. Bring the water to a boil over high heat. Add the asparagus to the steamer, cover, and cook until crisp-tender, about 4 minutes. Remove the asparagus, and run it under cold water to stop the cooking.

2. Place the roast beef slices on a work surface, and roll 1 asparagus spear inside 1 slice of roast beef. Repeat until all the slices are filled.

3. In a small bowl, whisk the vinegar with mustard. Dip the roll-ups in the dressing.

Nut-free

RELEASE

Lunch

PER SERVING
CALORIES: 231
CARBS: 3G
FAT: 7G
PROTEIN: 36G
SUGAR: 1G

Jicama Sticks with Chili and Lime

SERVES 6 / PREP TIME: 5 MINUTES

Jicama is the tuberous root of a native Mexican vine in the bean family. It has a very neutral flavor, along with a crunch like carrots. Here, a squeeze of lime and a dash of chili make a satisfying appetizer or snack.

Time-saving tip: *You can buy precut jicama in many grocery stores and salad bars. However, you will need to use the jicama within two or three days, because it won't stay fresh for long once it's cut.*

1 large jicama, peeled and cut into sticks
Juice of ½ lime
¼ teaspoon chili powder

1. Lay the jicama on a plate.
2. Squeeze the lime juice over the jicama.
3. Sprinkle with the chili powder and serve.

Nut-free
Paleo-friendly
Vegan

RELEASE

Snacks

PER SERVING
CALORIES: 56
CARBS: 16G
FAT: 0G
PROTEIN: 1G
SUGAR: 4G

Zucchini Chips

SERVES 2 / PREP TIME: 10 MINUTES / COOK TIME: 2 HOURS

Fried chips are wonderful for dips like salsa and hummus, but they often contain unhealthy ingredients and a lot of fat. These baked zucchini chips can stand in for grain-based, higher-fat, higher-carbohydrate chips, and they're still crispy and delicious. For the crispiest chips, allow them to cool completely before you eat them.

Technique tip: *Salting the zucchini before cooking and allowing it to sit in a colander draws the water out, making for a crispier chip.*

1 zucchini, cut into ⅛-inch slices
½ teaspoon sea salt, plus more for salting
¼ teaspoon freshly ground black pepper
½ teaspoon paprika
1 tablespoon extra-virgin olive oil

Nut-free
Paleo-friendly
Vegan

RELEASE

Snacks

PER SERVING
CALORIES: 78
CARBS: 4G
FAT: 7G
PROTEIN: 1G
SUGAR: 2G

1. Preheat the oven to 225°F. Line a rimmed baking pan with parchment paper.
2. Put the zucchini slices in a colander, and sprinkle them with salt, making sure each slice is salted. Let the zucchini slices sit for about 10 minutes.
3. Blot the zucchini with a paper towel, wiping away all moisture and salt.
4. In a small bowl, combine ½ teaspoon salt, pepper, and paprika. Toss the zucchini slices with the salt, pepper, and paprika mixture. Add the olive oil and toss again.
5. Put the zucchini slices in a single layer on the prepared baking sheet.
6. Put the chips in the oven and bake until crispy, about 2 hours.

Garlic Kale Chips

SERVES 2 / PREP TIME: 5 MINUTES / COOK TIME: 45 MINUTES

Bake up a big batch of these lightly crispy kale chips on the weekend, and store them in a tightly sealed container. The chips will last up to five days. While kale chips aren't sturdy enough to hold up to dip, they are lightly crispy, with a satisfying brittleness that shatters when you bite them.

Ingredient tip: *For a cheesy flavor, add about 2 tablespoons of nutritional yeast to the garlic powder and salt. Nutritional yeast is deactivated yeast flakes; find it at your local health food store. Use this ingredient in moderation because it is relatively high in carbs, at 4 grams per tablespoon.*

Nut-free
Paleo-friendly
Vegan

RELEASE

Snacks

PER SERVING
CALORIES: 171
CARBS: 11G
FAT: 14G
PROTEIN: 3G
SUGAR: 0G

1 bunch curly kale, torn into bite-size pieces
2 tablespoons extra-virgin olive oil
½ teaspoon sea salt
¼ teaspoon garlic powder

1. Preheat the oven to 200°F. Line a rimmed baking sheet with parchment paper.

2. In a large bowl, toss together the kale and olive oil.

3. In a small bowl, mix the salt and garlic powder. Toss with the kale and olive oil.

4. Put the kale in a single layer on the prepared baking sheet. Bake until the kale is dry and crisp, about 45 minutes (or longer for thicker pieces).

Daikon Radish Fries

SERVES 2 / PREP TIME: 10 MINUTES / COOK TIME: 20 MINUTES

If you're craving French fries but don't want the fat or carbohydrates, what do you do? These daikon radish fries are a great solution. Lower in carbs than potatoes, the daikon radishes are baked with a little bit of olive oil and sea salt to a delicious golden brown. If you have a mandoline, use it to cut the radishes into a perfect fry-size julienne.

2 daikon radishes, peeled and cut into 3-by-½-inch julienne

2 tablespoons extra-virgin olive oil

½ teaspoon sea salt, plus more for sprinkling

1. Preheat the oven to 475°F. Line a rimmed baking sheet with parchment paper.

2. In a colander, rinse the peeled and cut radishes. Drain the radishes, and pat them dry. Put them in a large bowl.

3. Add the olive oil and salt to the bowl. Toss to coat the radishes.

4. Put the radishes on the prepared baking sheet in a single layer. Bake until they are golden, about 15 to 20 minutes.

5. Sprinkle with additional sea salt, if you wish.

Nut-free
Paleo-friendly
Vegan

RELEASE

Snacks

PER SERVING
CALORIES: 121
CARBS: 1G
FAT: 14G
PROTEIN: 0G
SUGAR: 0G

Cauliflower "Popcorn"

SERVES 2 / PREP TIME: 15 MINUTES / COOK TIME: 30 MINUTES

Popcorn is a favorite snack, but it is high in carbs. Roasted cauliflower is a low-carb replacement that is equally delicious and easy to eat. To make this snack crispy, break the cauliflower into popcorn-size florets and trim away any excess stems. Then enjoy it hot by the handful the next time you crave popcorn.

3 cups small cauliflower florets

2 tablespoons extra-virgin olive oil

½ teaspoon sea salt

½ teaspoon garlic powder

Nut-free
Paleo-friendly
Vegan

RELEASE

Snacks

PER SERVING
CALORIES: 160
CARBS: 9G
FAT: 14G
PROTEIN: 3G
SUGAR: 4G

1. Preheat the oven to 400°F. Line a rimmed baking sheet with parchment paper.

2. In a medium bowl, toss the cauliflower with the olive oil, salt, and garlic powder.

3. Spread the cauliflower in a single layer on the prepared baking sheet.

4. Bake until the cauliflower is golden, 25 to 30 minutes.

Hardboiled Egg Whites with Garlicky Squash Purée

SERVES 6 / PREP TIME: 20 MINUTES, PLUS 2 HOURS TO CHILL /
COOK TIME: 20 MINUTES

Egg whites are filled with protein, while the yolks all contain the fat. These handy bite-size snacks give you the delicious protein without the fat. The flavor comes from a tasty roasted garlic and zucchini purée.

Technique tip: *This recipe calls for roasted garlic, which you can get in the deli section of many grocery stores. If you'd like to roast your own garlic, it's easy to do. Cut the tops off of two heads of garlic, exposing the cloves. Put the garlic in a bread pan, drizzle with olive oil, and sprinkle with sea salt. Cover the pan with foil, and roast the garlic in a 350°F oven for 90 minutes, until the garlic is soft and golden. To get the cloves out of the papery skin, simply squeeze the entire bulb of garlic over a bowl.*

6 hardboiled eggs, chilled and peeled

2 tablespoons extra-virgin olive oil

2 cups diced zucchini

8 roasted garlic cloves

Zest and juice of ½ lemon

¼ teaspoon sea salt

¼ teaspoon freshly ground black pepper

Smoked paprika

2 tablespoons chopped fresh chives

1. Cut the eggs in half the long way. Carefully scoop out the yolks, and reserve for another use. Place the whites, cut side up, on a plate and set aside.

2. In a large sauté pan, heat the olive oil over medium-high heat until it shimmers.

3. Add the zucchini and cook, stirring occasionally, until it is very soft, about 10 minutes. »

Nut-free
Paleo-friendly
Vegetarian

RELEASE

Snacks

PER SERVING
CALORIES: 69
CARBS: 3G
FAT: 5G
PROTEIN: 4G
SUGAR: 1G

Hardboiled Egg Whites with Garlicky Squash Purée *continued*

4. In the bowl of a food processor fitted with a metal chopping blade, add the zucchini, roasted garlic, lemon zest and juice, salt, and pepper. Process until smooth. Or spread the mixture out on a large cutting board, and chop until the consistency is like egg salad.

5. Spoon the zucchini mixture into the prepared egg whites. Top with a sprinkle of smoked paprika and the chopped chives. Refrigerate for about 2 hours to chill before serving.

RELEASE

Snacks

Spicy Pumpkin Seeds

SERVES 8 / PREP TIME: 10 MINUTES / COOK TIME: 1 HOUR

Baking pumpkin seeds is a fall tradition for many families. And these delicious and crunchy seeds pack powerful nutrition. The seeds contain healthy omega-3 fatty acids, along with iron and magnesium. They are also a healthy source of dietary fiber—¼ cup of them contains 4 grams of fiber and just 6 grams of fat.

½ teaspoon sea salt

¼ teaspoon freshly ground black pepper

Dash of cayenne pepper

¼ teaspoon garlic powder

¼ teaspoon onion powder

¼ teaspoon chipotle chili powder

2 cups raw pumpkin seeds

2 tablespoons extra-virgin olive oil

1. Preheat the oven to 275°F. Line a rimmed baking sheet with parchment paper.

2. In a small bowl, combine the salt, pepper, cayenne, garlic powder, onion powder, and chipotle powder, mixing well.

3. In a medium bowl, combine the pumpkin seeds, olive oil, and spice blend. Toss to coat the seeds.

4. Spread the seeds in a single layer on the prepared baking sheet, and bake until the seeds are dry, about 1 hour.

Nut-free
Paleo-friendly
Vegan

RELEASE

Snacks

PER SERVING
CALORIES: 218
CARBS: 6G
FAT: 20G
PROTEIN: 8G
SUGAR: 0G

Lemony Tuna and Radishes

SERVES 2 / PREP TIME: 5 MINUTES

Perhaps because of their bitter flavor, radishes are often overlooked as a simple snack. Rich in folic acid, radishes pair beautifully with deep-flavored meats and fatty fish. They are also the perfect partner for canned tuna.

1 (5-ounce) can water-packed tuna, drained

6 radishes, minced

Juice of 1 lemon

½ teaspoon dried oregano

¼ teaspoon fine sea salt

4 large romaine lettuce leaves

Nut-free
Paleo-friendly

RELEASE

Snacks

PER SERVING
CALORIES: 106
CARBS: 2G
FAT: 1G
PROTEIN: 22G
SUGAR: 1G

1. In a small bowl, mix the tuna, radishes, lemon juice, oregano, and salt.

2. Divide the tuna mixture evenly among the lettuce leaves. Roll the leaves around the tuna to eat.

Salmon Cucumber Rounds

SERVES 4 / PREP TIME: 5 MINUTES

This dish is so easy to make and is really delicious. The cucumber rounds stand in for bread, making this a low-carb canapé. Bring it to your next potluck supper, and watch it disappear.

Substitution tip: *Replace the cucumber rounds with slices of yellow squash or zucchini for a different flavor and texture.*

1 cucumber, cut into ¼-inch rounds

1 teaspoon chopped fresh dill

4 ounces smoked salmon, cut into 1-inch squares

1 bunch fresh chives, minced

1. Place the cucumber rounds on a plate. Sprinkle with fresh dill.

2. Top each round with piece of salmon. Sprinkle with the chives.

Nut-free
Paleo-friendly

RELEASE

Snacks

PER SERVING
CALORIES: 46
CARBS: 3G
FAT: 1G
PROTEIN: 6G
SUGAR: 0G

Smoked Trout Wraps

SERVES 2 / PREP TIME: 5 MINUTES

Smoked trout has a lovely, rich flavor. The brining and smoking process is a preservative; keep it tightly sealed in the refrigerator for up to a couple of weeks. Because of its firm, fatty flesh, you can even freeze it.

4 ounces smoked trout, skinned and flaked

Zest and juice of 1 lemon

1 tablespoon capers

1 head Bibb (butterhead) lettuce, leaves separated

1 medium carrot, peeled and grated

Nut-free
Paleo-friendly

RELEASE

Snacks

PER SERVING
CALORIES: 126
CARBS: 4G
FAT: 1G
PROTEIN: 16G
SUGAR: 2G

1. In a small bowl, toss the trout with the lemon zest and juice, and capers.

2. Place 1 tablespoon of the trout mixture in each lettuce leaf. Top with the grated carrot.

Quick Pickled Cucumber and Turkey Roll-Ups

SERVES: 6 / PREP TIME: 30 MINUTES, PLUS 4 HOURS FOR PICKLING

If you slice cucumbers thinly enough, you can pickle them in the refrigerator in just a few hours. To slice the cucumbers for this recipe, cut them in ⅛- to ¼-inch slices along the length of the cucumber.

1 cup apple cider vinegar

1 cup red wine vinegar

2 garlic cloves, crushed

½ tablespoon sea salt

12 cucumber slices, ⅛-inch thick, cut along the length of the cucumber

12 slices gluten-free deli turkey

2 tablespoons Dijon mustard

2 tablespoons chopped fresh dill

Nut-free
Paleo-friendly

RELEASE

Snacks

PER SERVING
CALORIES: 139
CARBS: 11G
FAT: 3G
PROTEIN: 14G
SUGAR: 5G

1. In a medium bowl, whisk together the apple cider vinegar, red wine vinegar, garlic, and salt until well combined.

2. Add the cucumber, and submerge in the vinegar mixture. Cover with plastic wrap, and refrigerate at least 4 hours, or overnight, to allow the cucumber to pickle.

3. Remove the cucumber slices from the brine, and pat them dry. Put them on a platter.

4. On top of each cucumber slice, place a slice of deli turkey breast. Spread the turkey with mustard, and sprinkle it with chopped dill.

5. Roll the cucumber around the turkey, and secure the roll with a toothpick.

6. Refrigerate for up to 3 days or serve right away.

Ham, Basil, and Spinach Rolls

SERVES 2 / PREP TIME: 5 MINUTES

When purchasing any deli meat, ask at the deli counter to make sure you are not buying meat that contains gluten or sugar as part of the soaking solution.

Substitution tip: *You can replace the ham with any thinly sliced deli meat, such as roast beef, turkey, chicken, or turkey ham.*

6 thin slices deli ham

2 tablespoons Dijon mustard

12 baby spinach leaves

12 basil leaves

Nut-free
Paleo-friendly

RELEASE

Snacks

PER SERVING
CALORIES: 56
CARBS: 3G
FAT: 2G
PROTEIN: 7G
SUGAR: 0G

1. Spread each slice of ham with mustard.

2. Place 2 spinach leaves and 2 basil leaves on each slice of ham.

3. Roll the ham slices around the spinach and basil.

Egg Drop Soup

SERVES 4 / PREP TIME: 10 MINUTES / COOK TIME: 15 MINUTES

This vegetable soup has plenty of antioxidants, thanks to the kale and other vegetables. The egg whites add a bit of protein as well. You can store the soup in the refrigerator, tightly sealed, for up to 3 days.

Substitution tip: *If you like, you can replace the kale with baby spinach, Swiss chard, or some other dark leafy green. For a very colorful soup, remove the stems from the Swiss chard and cut them into a ¼-inch dice. Sauté the stems with the greens in step 2 until they soften. Then continue with the recipe as written.*

1 tablespoon olive oil

1 bunch kale, stems removed and leaves cut into ¼-inch ribbons

6 cups low-sodium chicken broth

6 scallions, thinly sliced

4 shiitake mushrooms, stemmed and sliced

1 carrot, peeled and cut into ¼-inch dice

½ cup frozen peas

1 teaspoon gluten-free soy sauce

Pinch of white pepper

4 egg whites

Nut-free

RELEASE

Dinner

PER SERVING
CALORIES: 147
CARBS: 20G
FAT: 4G
PROTEIN: 10G
SUGAR: 5G

1. In a large saucepan, heat the oil over medium-high heat until it shimmers. Add the kale, and cook until it softens, about 3 minutes.

2. Add the broth, and bring it to a simmer. Add the scallions, mushrooms, and carrot. Simmer until the carrots are soft, about 4 minutes.

3. Stir in the peas, soy sauce, and white pepper. Cook for 3 minutes more to allow the flavors to blend.

4. In a small bowl, whisk the egg whites. Pour them into the simmering soup in a slow stream, stirring the soup with a fork as you do.

5. Cook for 1 minute more, until the egg whites create opaque ribbons. Serve hot.

Leafy Greens Soup

SERVES 4 / PREP TIME: 10 MINUTES / COOK TIME: 35 MINUTES

Southern versions of this dish often call for smoked sausage to balance out the tart flavor of the greens. Instead of meat, this recipe adds smoky heat in two ways—smoked paprika and dried chili. Look for both in the spice section of your local supermarket.

4¼ cups low-sodium vegetable broth, divided

1 onion, coarsely chopped

1 green bell pepper, seeded and chopped

1 pound chopped collards, mustard greens, or other dark, leafy greens

¼ cup apple cider vinegar

1 whole dried chili, such as chipotle

1½ tablespoons smoked paprika

½ teaspoon dried thyme

½ teaspoon freshly ground black pepper

¼ teaspoon salt

Nut-free
Vegan

RELEASE

Dinner

PER SERVING
CALORIES: 81
CARBS: 14G
FAT: 1G
PROTEIN: 6G
SUGAR: 4G

1. In a large, deep, nonstick saucepan, heat ¼ cup broth over medium-high heat. Add the onion, bell pepper, and greens, and stir to combine. If the vegetable mixture looks a bit dry, add another ¼ cup of liquid to moisten.

2. Cook, stirring frequently, until the onions begin to soften, about 5 minutes. Add the vinegar, stir to coat, and cook for 1 minute more.

3. Add the dried chili, paprika, thyme, pepper, and salt, and stir to combine. Cook for 2 minutes more.

4. Add the remaining 4 cups broth. Turn the heat to high, and bring the mixture to a boil. When the soup begins to boil, reduce the heat to a simmer. Cover and cook until the greens are tender, about 20 minutes.

Vegetable Soup with Clams and Greens

SERVES 4 / PREP TIME: 10 MINUTES / COOK TIME: 10 MINUTES

Littleneck clams are common on the East Coast and tend to be a bit bigger than Manila clams. To make this recipe, look for about a pound of your favorite type of clams.

Ingredient tip: *Wash the clams by soaking them in cold water for 20 minutes to remove any grit. Discard any clams with cracked, chipped, or broken shells.*

16 littleneck or 24 Manila clams (about 1 pound)

3 cups low-sodium vegetable broth

¼ teaspoon Old Bay seasoning

1 tablespoon arrowroot powder

2 cups baby spinach leaves

2 cups baby kale leaves

2 carrots, peeled and grated

3 tablespoons thinly sliced scallions

Nut-free

RELEASE

Dinner

PER SERVING
CALORIES: 97
CARBS: 12G
FAT: 1G
PROTEIN: 11G
SUGAR: 2G

1. Bring a large pot of water to a boil over high heat. Add the clams and return to a boil. Reduce the heat to medium, cover, and cook until the clams open, 4 to 6 minutes. Drain the clams into a colander. Rinse any grit out of the pot.

2. Add the broth to the pot, and bring to a simmer over medium-high heat.

3. Meanwhile, remove the clam meat from the shells. Discard the shells and any unopened clams. Divide the clam meat among 4 bowls.

4. Add the Old Bay seasoning and the arrowroot powder to the broth, and stir to combine. Stir in the spinach, kale, and carrots. Cook until the spinach wilts, about 1 minute.

5. Ladle the hot broth and greens over the clams. Garnish with the scallions, and serve immediately.

Slow Cooker Turkey Meatball Soup with Kale

SERVES 6 / PREP TIME: 30 MINUTES / COOK TIME: 4 TO 10 HOURS IN A SLOW COOKER

Set your slow cooker on high in the afternoon, and this very hearty soup/stew will be ready by dinnertime. Or make it overnight and reheat it in the evening. Either way, this dish will nourish you with rich meatballs, a delicious broth, and plenty of veggies. It keeps well in the freezer for up to six months. Make a double batch, and you'll have plenty for lunches as well as dinners.

Nut-free

RELEASE

Dinner

PER SERVING
CALORIES: 219
CARBS: 8G
FAT: 10G
PROTEIN: 27G
SUGAR: 3G

For the meatballs

1 pound ground turkey

3 garlic cloves, finely minced

1 cup baby spinach, chopped into small pieces

1 teaspoon sea salt

¼ teaspoon freshly ground black pepper

1 teaspoon dried thyme

Pinch of red pepper flakes

½ teaspoon Dijon mustard

For the soup

6 cups low-sodium chicken broth

1 onion, chopped

4 garlic cloves chopped

2 carrots, peeled and sliced

2 celery stalks, sliced

1 zucchini, chopped

1 teaspoon dried thyme

1 cup chopped kale

Sea salt

Freshly ground black pepper

To make the meatballs

1. In a large bowl, combine the turkey, garlic, spinach, salt, pepper, thyme, red pepper flakes, and mustard. Mix with your hands to incorporate all the ingredients.

2. Roll the turkey mixture into 1-inch meatballs, and put them in a slow cooker.

To make the soup

1. Add the broth, onion, garlic, carrots, celery, zucchini, and thyme to the slow cooker along with the meatballs.

2. Cover the slow cooker, and cook on high for 4 to 5 hours or low for 8 to 10 hours, until the meatballs are cooked through.

3. In the last hour of cooking, stir in the kale. Cook for one more hour.

4. Season with salt and pepper.

RELEASE

Dinner

Roasted Portobello Mushrooms with Garlic-Cauliflower Mash

SERVES 4 / PREP TIME: 15 MINUTES / COOK TIME: 20 MINUTES

Portobello mushrooms have a deep, savory flavor. The large mushrooms roast up beautifully and are very filling. Serve these mushrooms with a garlic-scented cauliflower purée reminiscent of mashed potatoes—without all the carbs or fat.

Technique tip: *Don't submerge mushrooms in water, because they soak it up like a sponge, yielding mushy mushrooms. To clean the mushrooms, gently wipe away dirt with a paper towel. Remove the gills and stem of the portobello mushrooms before cooking by scraping the edge of a spoon along the underside of the mushroom. Discard the gills.*

Paleo-friendly
Vegan

RELEASE

Dinner

PER SERVING
CALORIES: 108
CARBS: 9G
FAT: 7G
PROTEIN: 5G
SUGAR: 2G

2 tablespoons olive oil

½ teaspoon garlic salt

1 teaspoon freshly ground black pepper, divided

4 large portobello mushrooms, stems and gills removed

1 head cauliflower, broken into florets

6 roasted garlic cloves (jarred or homemade)

¼ cup unsweetened, unflavored almond milk

½ teaspoon fine sea salt

2 tablespoons chopped fresh chives

1. Preheat the oven to 400°F. Line a baking sheet with parchment paper.

2. Whisk together the oil, garlic salt, and ½ teaspoon pepper. Brush the mixture onto both sides of the mushrooms.

3. Place the mushrooms on the lined baking sheet, and bake until browned on one side, about 10 minutes. Flip the mushrooms, and continue baking for an additional 10 minutes.

4. Meanwhile, place a steamer in a large saucepan, and add water to a level just below the bottom of the steamer. Bring to a boil over high heat. Add the cauliflower to the steamer, cover, and cook until soft, about 10 minutes.

5. In the bowl of a food processor, process the steamed cauliflower, roasted garlic cloves, almond milk, sea salt, and remaining $\frac{1}{2}$ teaspoon pepper until smooth. Or mash by hand in a large bowl with a potato masher, or use an immersion blender to mash and blend the cauliflower. Taste and adjust the seasonings if necessary.

6. Sprinkle the cauliflower with the chopped fresh chives, and serve alongside the roasted portobello mushrooms.

Shiitake Fajitas

SERVES 4 / PREP TIME: 10 MINUTES / COOK TIME: 10 MINUTES

Shiitake mushrooms replace meat in these tasty fajitas. Shiitakes are high in fiber and iron. Clean the mushrooms by gently wiping them with a paper towel or using a soft mushroom brush. Serve the fajitas wrapped in lettuce leaves and topped with pico de gallo.

2 tablespoons olive oil

16 ounces shiitake mushrooms, stemmed and sliced

1 onion, sliced

1 green bell pepper, seeded and sliced

3 garlic cloves, minced

Juice of 3 limes

1 teaspoon chipotle chili powder

½ teaspoon ground cumin

½ teaspoon fine sea salt

Pinch of cayenne pepper

8 large green lettuce leaves

1 cup pico de gallo (see Breakfast Tacos, page 151)

Nut-free
Paleo-friendly
Vegan

RELEASE

Dinner

PER SERVING
CALORIES: 197
CARBS: 27G
FAT: 7G
PROTEIN: 4G
SUGAR: 9G

1. In a large sauté pan, heat the olive oil over medium-high heat until it shimmers. Add the mushrooms, onion, and bell pepper. Cook, stirring occasionally, until the vegetables are soft and begin to brown, about 7 minutes.

2. Add the garlic and cook, stirring constantly, until it is fragrant, about 30 seconds.

3. In a small bowl, whisk together the lime juice, chipotle powder, cumin, salt, and cayenne. Pour over the vegetables. Cook, stirring constantly, until the sauce thickens slightly, about 2 minutes. Scrape any browned bits from the bottom of the pan with a spoon.

4. Spoon the mushroom mixture onto the lettuce leaves. Serve the fajitas topped with pico de gallo.

Crustless Broccoli and Mushroom Quiche

SERVES 4 / PREP TIME: 10 MINUTES / COOK TIME: 35 MINUTES

Eggs are an excellent source of protein. This recipe uses eggs as a protein binder and then adds tasty mushrooms and broccoli. The fat content is kept low by replacing some of the whole eggs with egg whites.

Nonstick cooking spray

1 tablespoon olive oil

1 onion, chopped

8 ounces shiitake mushrooms, stemmed and sliced

1 cup broccoli florets

2 garlic cloves, minced

4 whole eggs

4 egg whites

½ cup unsweetened, unflavored almond milk

½ teaspoon fine sea salt

¼ teaspoon freshly ground black pepper

Dash of cayenne pepper

**Paleo-friendly
Vegetarian**

RELEASE

Dinner

PER SERVING
CALORIES: 165
CARBS: 13G
FAT: 9G
PROTEIN: 11G
SUGAR: 4G

1. Preheat the oven to 375°F. Spray a 9-inch pie pan with nonstick cooking spray.

2. In a large sauté pan, heat the olive oil over medium-high heat until it shimmers. Add the onion, mushrooms, and broccoli, and cook, stirring occasionally, until the vegetables begin to soften, about 6 minutes.

3. Add the garlic and cook, stirring constantly, until the garlic is fragrant, about 30 seconds. Spoon the vegetables into the prepared pie pan.

4. In a medium bowl, whisk together the whole eggs, egg whites, almond milk, salt, pepper, and cayenne. Carefully pour the egg mixture over the vegetables in the pie pan.

5. Bake until the quiche is set, about 25 minutes. Cut into wedges and serve.

Lemony Mussels with Green Beans, Fennel, and Red Bell Pepper

SERVES 4 / PREP TIME: 10 MINUTES / COOK TIME: 15 MINUTES

This brothy dish features mussels and bright lemon flavors, along with crisp green beans and red bell peppers. Carefully pick over and clean the mussels before using them, and be sure to discard any that are cracked or open.

2 tablespoons olive oil

1 onion, finely chopped

1 fennel bulb, diced

1 red bell pepper, seeded and chopped

½ pound green beans, cut into 1-inch pieces

3 garlic cloves, minced

Juice of 2 lemons

Zest of 1 lemon

2 cups low-sodium chicken broth

2 pounds fresh mussels

Fine sea salt

Freshly ground black pepper

2 tablespoons minced fennel fronds

Nut-free

RELEASE

Dinner

PER SERVING
CALORIES: 323
CARBS: 22G
FAT: 14G
PROTEIN: 30G
SUGAR: 3G

1. In a large sauté pan, heat the olive oil over medium-high heat until it shimmers. Add the onion, fennel bulb, bell pepper, and green beans, and cook, stirring occasionally, until the vegetables soften and begin to brown, about 7 minutes.

2. Add the garlic and cook, stirring constantly, until it is fragrant, about 30 seconds.

3. Add the lemon juice, lemon zest, broth, and mussels. Cover and simmer until the mussels open, about 5 minutes. Discard any mussels that did not open.

4. Season with salt and pepper. Stir in the fennel fronds just before serving.

Shrimp with Okra and Bell Pepper

SERVES 4 / PREP TIME: 10 MINUTES / COOK TIME: 30 MINUTES

Serve this for dinner, and then turn the leftovers into a salad for lunch the next day. Chill the salad in portion-size containers and grab one on your way out the door in the morning. You can find okra in the produce or freezer section of the grocery store.

Time-saving tip: *When the weather is warm and you don't want to turn on the oven, or you're just in a hurry, stir-fry the vegetables instead. Okra should be seared in a very hot pan and cooked quickly. Make sure there is no extra moisture in the pan when stir-frying, or the okra will get soggy.*

2 cups fresh or frozen okra, halved

1 medium onion, diced

1 red bell pepper, seeded and cut into ½-inch pieces

1¾ teaspoons Old Bay seasoning, divided

1 pound uncooked large shrimp, peeled and deveined

1 tablespoon olive oil

1. Preheat the oven to 400°F. Line a rimmed baking sheet with parchment paper.

2. Spread the okra, onion, and bell pepper in a single layer on the baking sheet, and sprinkle with ¾ teaspoon Old Bay seasoning. Roast the vegetables, stirring occasionally, until tender, 20 to 25 minutes.

3. Meanwhile, sprinkle the shrimp with the remaining 1 teaspoon Old Bay seasoning. Heat the oil in a large nonstick skillet over medium-high heat until it shimmers. Add the shrimp and cook, 1 minute per side, until it is pink and opaque.

4. Toss the shrimp with the vegetables and serve.

Nut-free
Paleo-friendly

RELEASE

Dinner

PER SERVING
CALORIES: 159
CARBS: 10G
FAT: 4G
PROTEIN: 23G
SUGAR: 3G

Spinach-Stuffed Fillet of Sole with Green Beans

SERVES 4 / PREP TIME: 10 MINUTES / COOK TIME: 30 MINUTES

This recipe serves up a double helping of healthy green vegetables. Fillet of sole is a relatively mild and low-fat fish. If you'd like, you can replace it with any other white fish, or with trout. Choose fish with firm flesh that has a clean, salty (but not fishy) scent. You can also substitute frozen spinach and green beans in this recipe for fresh, if you wish.

1 pound green beans, trimmed

2 tablespoons olive oil, divided

⅓ cup chopped celery

6 scallions, minced

2 tablespoons chopped fresh dill

½ cup chopped fresh baby spinach

Juice of 1 lemon

Zest of ½ lemon

½ teaspoon fine sea salt, divided

¼ teaspoon freshly ground black pepper

Nonstick cooking spray

1 pound sole fillets

¼ cup low-sodium vegetable broth

1. Preheat the oven to 350°F.

2. Place a steamer in a large saucepan, and add water to a level just below the bottom of the steamer. Bring the water to a boil over high heat. Add the green beans to the steamer, cover, and steam until crisp-tender, 4 to 5 minutes. Remove the beans, and run them under cold water to stop the cooking. Drain and reserve.

3. Heat 1 tablespoon olive oil in a small nonstick skillet over medium heat. Add the celery, and sauté until softened, 3 to 5 minutes. Turn off the stove. Add the scallions, dill, spinach, lemon juice, lemon zest, ¼ teaspoon salt, and the pepper to the warm pan, and stir to combine.

4. Lightly spray a 9-inch square baking dish with nonstick cooking spray. Arrange half the sole fillets in a single layer in the baking dish. Sprinkle the vegetable mixture over the fillets, and place the remaining fillets over the top. Add the broth to the pan, and cover the dish with aluminum foil. Bake until the fish is opaque, 15 to 20 minutes.

5. In a nonstick sauté pan, heat the remaining 1 tablespoon oil over medium-high heat. Add the green beans and the remaining ¼ teaspoon salt. Cook until the beans are tender, about 4 minutes. Serve with the sole.

RELEASE

Dinner

Grilled Salmon and Green Beans with Mustard and Thyme

SERVES 4 / PREP TIME: 20 MINUTES (INCLUDES MARINATING TIME) / COOK TIME: 20 MINUTES

While fresh salmon is preferable in this recipe, you can use frozen salmon. Cook the fish with its skin on to preserve flavor and moisture. However, the skin is too fatty for this stage of the diet, so remove it before serving.

1 pound green beans, trimmed

Zest and juice of 1 lemon

1 tablespoon coarse-grain mustard

1 teaspoon dried thyme

1 (1-pound) salmon fillet, with skin on

1 tablespoon olive oil

Sea salt

Freshly ground black pepper

Nut-free
Paleo-friendly

RELEASE

Dinner

PER SERVING
CALORIES: 179
CARBS: 9G
FAT: 6G
PROTEIN: 25G
SUGAR: 3G

1. Place a steamer in a large saucepan, and add water to a level just below the bottom of the steamer. Bring the water to a boil over high heat. Add the green beans, cover, and cook until still crisp, about 4 minutes. Remove the beans, and run them under cold water to stop the cooking. Set aside.

2. In a small bowl, combine the lemon zest and juice, mustard, and thyme. Pour half the mixture into a shallow dish, and add the salmon, flesh-side down. Leave it to marinate for 10 minutes.

3. In a large cast iron pan, heat the olive oil over medium-high heat until it shimmers. Add the green beans and cook, stirring occasionally, until tender, 3 to 4 minutes. Remove the beans from the pan, and put them in a serving bowl. Add the remaining half of the mustard mixture to the beans. Toss to coat. Season with salt and pepper.

4. Add the salmon to the pan, flesh-side down, and cook for 1 minute. Carefully flip the fish over, and cook for an additional 6 minutes. Serve the salmon with the green beans.

Halibut Niçoise

SERVES 4 / PREP TIME: 30 MINUTES (INCLUDES MARINATING TIME) /
COOK TIME: 15 MINUTES

This recipe is a variation of the well-known salade Niçoise. *This salad typically contains tuna, which is replaced here with halibut, a fish that has less fat. The traditional high-carb potatoes are also omitted from this version.*

Substitution tip: *If you can't find Niçoise olives, you can use any red or green olives. Many grocery stores have an olive bar in the deli section or a selection of olives in the salad bar.*

¼ cup white wine vinegar

1 tablespoon Dijon mustard

1 garlic clove, minced

¾ teaspoon fine sea salt, divided

Zest and juice of 1 lemon

1 pound halibut fillets

Freshly ground black pepper

2 tablespoons olive oil

1 large head Bibb (butterhead) lettuce, separated into leaves

8 ounces sugar-free pickled green beans or other pickled vegetable, drained

1½ cups grape tomatoes, halved

3 hardboiled eggs, peeled and quartered

¼ cup pitted Niçoise olives

¼ cup finely chopped fresh flat-leaf parsley

Nut-free
Paleo-friendly

RELEASE

Dinner

PER SERVING
CALORIES: 298
CARBS: 9G
FAT: 14G
PROTEIN: 29G
SUGAR: 4G

1. In a small bowl, whisk together the vinegar, mustard, garlic, and ¼ teaspoon salt until well blended. Set aside.

2. Combine the lemon zest and juice with ¼ teaspoon salt in a sturdy zip-top plastic bag. Add the halibut, and marinate for 20 minutes. Drain the fish, and season with the remaining ¼ teaspoon salt and the pepper. »

Halibut Niçoise *continued*

3. In a cast iron skillet, heat the olive oil over medium-high heat until it shimmers. Add the fish to the pan, flesh side down, and cook until just browned, about 1 minute. Carefully flip the fish over, and cook until the flesh is no longer translucent, about 10 minutes more. Remove from the heat and flake.

4. On a large platter, place the lettuce in a single layer. Add the pickled vegetables, tomatoes, eggs, olives, and fish. Sprinkle with the parsley.

5. Drizzle with the dressing and serve.

RELEASE

Dinner

Poached Chicken and Mixed Vegetables

SERVES 4 / PREP TIME: 10 MINUTES / COOK TIME: 10 MINUTES

This dish works beautifully—and quickly—with the frozen packages of precut stir-fry vegetables that are available at most supermarkets. Choose a package that has broccoli and ingredients such as red peppers and onions.

½ cup low-sodium vegetable broth

2 garlic cloves, minced

1 tablespoon minced fresh ginger

1 tablespoon gluten-free soy sauce

1 (15-ounce) bag frozen mixed stir-fry vegetables

1 pound chicken breast tenders, cut into 1-inch pieces

Fine sea salt

Freshly ground black pepper

2 scallions, minced

1. In a large saucepan, heat the broth over medium-high heat until it just starts to simmer. Add the garlic, ginger, and soy sauce to the pan, and stir to combine.

2. Add the frozen vegetables and cook, stirring occasionally, until they are cooked through, about 5 minutes. Transfer the vegetables to a large bowl using a slotted spoon.

3. Sprinkle the chicken with salt and pepper. Add the chicken to the broth mixture, and cook, stirring occasionally, until it is cooked through, about 5 minutes.

4. Remove the chicken from the broth, and add it to the bowl with the cooked vegetables. Serve garnished with the scallions.

Nut-free

RELEASE

Dinner

PER SERVING
CALORIES: 154
CARBS: 7G
FAT: 1G
PROTEIN: 26G
SUGAR: 0G

Curry Chicken with Cauliflower

SERVES 4 / PREP TIME: 20 MINUTES, PLUS 1 HOUR TO MARINATE /
COOK TIME: 30 MINUTES

This recipe can easily be doubled, with the leftovers frozen and used for quick lunches or dinners later in the month. Break the cauliflower into small florets so it cooks through quickly in the oven. If you don't like cilantro, you can omit it or substitute flat-leaf parsley.

Nut-free
Paleo-friendly

RELEASE

Dinner

PER SERVING
CALORIES: 241
CARBS: 6G
FAT: 8G
PROTEIN: 35G
SUGAR: 2G

¼ cup plus 1 tablespoon olive oil, divided

Juice of 1 lemon

1 garlic clove, minced

1 teaspoon curry powder

1 teaspoon ground coriander

1 teaspoon ground ginger

¾ teaspoon fine sea salt, divided

¼ teaspoon cayenne pepper

1½ pounds chicken breast tenders

1 small head cauliflower, cut into florets

1 small onion, quartered

Freshly ground black pepper

¼ cup chopped fresh cilantro

1. In a shallow glass dish, combine ¼ cup olive oil, the lemon juice, garlic, curry powder, coriander, ginger, ½ teaspoon salt, and the cayenne. Add the chicken and turn to coat. Cover and marinate in the refrigerator for 1 hour.

2. Preheat the oven to 450°F. Line a large rimmed baking sheet with parchment paper. Remove the chicken from the marinade, and arrange pieces on the prepared baking sheet. Discard the marinade.

3. In a medium bowl, toss the cauliflower and onion with the remaining 1 tablespoon olive oil, and add it to the baking sheet. Season the vegetables with the remaining ¼ teaspoon salt and pepper.

4. Roast the chicken and vegetables for 30 minutes, turning the chicken and stirring the vegetables halfway through. Serve garnished with the cilantro.

Chicken Thighs with Swiss Chard

SERVES 4 / PREP TIME: 10 MINUTES / COOK TIME: 45 MINUTES

To give a bit more kick to this recipe, add ¼ cup red wine vinegar to the pan when you add the chicken broth. The acidity will balance the bitter flavor of the Swiss chard. If you like a bit of spice, you can also add ¼ teaspoon red pepper flakes.

Ingredient tip: *Bright and colorful Swiss chard stems can add a pop of color to the dish. If you'd like to include the stems in the dish, cut them into small pieces and sauté them in a little olive oil until they are soft, about 6 minutes.*

2 tablespoons olive oil, divided

1½ pounds boneless, skinless chicken thighs

Fine sea salt

Freshly ground black pepper

½ teaspoon dried thyme

½ teaspoon garlic powder

1 bunch Swiss chard, stems removed, leaves chopped

2 garlic cloves, sliced

½ medium onion, coarsely chopped

1½ cups low-sodium chicken broth

1. Preheat the oven to 350°F.

2. In a large, nonstick sauté pan, heat 1 tablespoon olive oil over medium-high heat until it shimmers. Sprinkle the chicken with salt, pepper, thyme, and garlic powder.

3. Add the chicken to the pan, and cook until it is brown on the bottom, about 6 minutes. Turn the chicken over, and cook until the other side is brown, about 6 minutes more. Remove the chicken from the pan.

4. Add the remaining 1 tablespoon oil to the pan. Add the chard, garlic, and onion, and sauté, stirring occasionally, until the chard begins to wilt and soften, about 5 minutes. Add the broth to the pan, and bring it to a simmer. Return the chicken to the pan, nestling it in among the chard leaves.

5. Cover the pan, and put it in the oven. Bake until the chicken is cooked through, about 25 minutes.

Nut-free

RELEASE

Dinner

PER SERVING
CALORIES: 400
CARBS: 3G
FAT: 20G
PROTEIN: 50G
SUGAR: 1G

Turkey Lettuce Cups

SERVES 4 / PREP TIME: 15 MINUTES / COOK TIME: 15 MINUTES

This dish combines classic Asian flavors such as garlic, ginger, sesame oil, and soy sauce with ground turkey and vegetables to make a high-protein, high-fiber meal. You can also serve the ground turkey mixture on a bed of spinach or other nutritious dark greens.

Substitution tip: *You can replace the ground turkey with ground chicken or lean ground pork. You can also swap out any of the vegetables called for with other vegetables you might enjoy, such as leafy greens or bell peppers. If you can't find shiitake mushrooms, substitute crimini mushrooms or button mushrooms.*

Nut-free

RELEASE

Dinner

PER SERVING
CALORIES: 436
CARBS: 47G
FAT: 12G
PROTEIN: 39G
SUGAR: 8G

2 teaspoons sesame oil

1 pound ground turkey

1 tablespoon grated fresh ginger

8 shiitake mushrooms, thinly sliced

1 (8-ounce) can water chestnuts, drained and chopped

4 scallions, minced

1 cup sugar snap peas, cut into 1-inch pieces

1 garlic clove, minced

½ cup low-sodium chicken broth

2 tablespoons gluten-free soy sauce

8 large romaine lettuce leaves

½ cup chopped fresh cilantro

1 large carrot, peeled and shredded

1. In a large nonstick pan, heat the sesame oil over medium-high heat until it shimmers. Add the turkey and cook, crumbling the meat, until it is browned, about 5 minutes. Remove the turkey from the oil with a slotted spoon, and set aside.

2. Add the ginger, mushrooms, water chestnuts, scallions, and snap peas to the hot pan. Cook, stirring occasionally, until the vegetables are crisp-tender, about 4 minutes. Add the garlic, and cook until it is fragrant, about 30 seconds.

3. Add the broth and soy sauce to the pan, scraping up any browned bits from the bottom of the pan. Return the cooked turkey to the pan. Stir to mix, and cook until the turkey is warmed through, about 2 minutes.

4. To serve, put 2 lettuce leaves on each place. Spoon the turkey mixture into the lettuce leaves, and top with cilantro and carrot.

RELEASE

Dinner

Turkey Scaloppini with Spinach

SERVES 4 / PREP TIME: 10 MINUTES / COOK TIME: 20 MINUTES

Pounding turkey into thin fillets, and giving them a quick sear in a pan really shortens the time it takes to cook turkey breasts. This scaloppini is rolled around a flavorful filling of sautéed spinach and then sliced for a pretty presentation.

4 (4-ounce) turkey breast cutlets

Fine sea salt

Freshly ground black pepper

2 tablespoons olive oil, divided

1 shallot, minced

9 ounces fresh baby spinach

3 garlic cloves, minced

Juice of 1 orange

Zest of ½ orange

Dash red pepper flakes

Nut-free
Paleo-friendly

RELEASE

Dinner

PER SERVING
CALORIES: 215
CARBS: 7G
FAT: 8G
PROTEIN: 30G
SUGAR: 2G

1. Put the turkey cutlets between two pieces of plastic wrap, and use a meat mallet or a rolling pin to pound them to ¼- to ½-inch thick. Season liberally with salt and pepper.

2. In a large nonstick skillet, heat 1 tablespoon olive oil over medium-high heat until it shimmers. Add the turkey and cook until it is opaque and cooked through, about 3 minutes per side. Remove the turkey from the pan, and set it aside on a platter.

3. Add the remaining 1 tablespoon olive oil to the pan, and heat until it shimmers. Add the shallot and cook until it is soft and begins to brown, about 6 minutes. Add the spinach, and cook until it wilts, about 2 minutes. Add the garlic, and cook until it is fragrant, about 30 seconds.

4. Add the orange juice, orange zest, and red pepper flakes. Cook, stirring frequently, until the liquid evaporates, about 3 minutes more.

5. Divide the spinach in equal parts among the turkey cutlets. Roll the turkey around the spinach, slice into rounds, and serve.

Zucchini Noodles with Meat Sauce

SERVES 4 / PREP TIME: 15 MINUTES / COOK TIME: 20 MINUTES

One popular way of replacing the carb- and gluten-laden spaghetti in pasta dishes is to substitute thinly sliced zucchini. You can make zucchini noodles by peeling the zucchini and using a vegetable peeler lengthwise along the zucchini to get long, thin strips. Then cut the strips into thinner strips. If that seems like too much work, you can buy a zucchini spiralizer, which cuts the zucchini for you.

Ingredient tip: *Some brands of tomato sauce and crushed tomatoes contain sugar. Read the labels carefully, and look for ones that don't list sugar, high-fructose corn syrup, or any other type of sweetener on the label.*

For the meat sauce

2 tablespoons olive oil

1 pound turkey Italian sausage, either bulk or removed from the casings

1 onion, chopped

1 cup sliced mushrooms

3 garlic cloves, minced

1 (14-ounce) can tomato sauce

1 (14-ounce) can crushed tomatoes, drained

1 teaspoon Italian seasoning

For the zucchini noodles

2 tablespoons olive oil

2 whole zucchini, peeled and cut into noodles

1 garlic clove, minced

¼ cup low-sodium chicken broth

Dash of salt

2 tablespoons chopped fresh basil

2 tablespoons chopped fresh flat-leaf parsley

To make the meat sauce

1. In a large pot, heat the olive oil over medium-high heat until it shimmers.

2. Add the Italian sausage and cook, crumbling with a spoon, until it is browned, about 7 minutes. »

Nut-free

RELEASE

Dinner

PER SERVING
CALORIES: 304
CARBS: 16G
FAT: 15G
PROTEIN: 26G
SUGAR: 10G

Zucchini Noodles with Meat Sauce *continued*

3. Add the onions and mushrooms, and cook, stirring occasionally, until the vegetables are soft, about 5 minutes more.

4. Add the garlic and cook, stirring constantly, until it is fragrant, about 30 seconds.

5. Add the tomato sauce, crushed tomatoes, and Italian seasoning, scraping any browned bits from the bottom of the pan.

6. Bring to a simmer, and reduce the heat to medium low. Simmer while you prepare the noodles.

To make the zucchini noodles

1. While the sauce simmers, in a large, nonstick sauté pan, heat the olive oil until it shimmers.

2. Add the zucchini and cook, stirring constantly, for 1 minute.

3. Add the garlic and cook, stirring constantly, for 30 seconds.

4. Add the broth and salt. Simmer until the zucchini softens, about 5 minutes more.

5. Drain the zucchini before serving.

6. Just before serving, toss the noodles with the sauce; then stir in the basil and parsley.

Slow Cooker Turkey Cabbage Rolls

SERVES 4 / PREP TIME: 20 MINUTES / COOK TIME: 4 TO 10 HOURS IN A SLOW COOKER

This recipe is a twist on both traditional cabbage rolls and pot stickers. Regular pot stickers contain gluten in the wraps. Making them into cabbage rolls gives you the flavor of pot stickers without the carbs. If you like cabbage rolls, you'll enjoy the Asian flair these have to offer. Avoid the sugar found in most store-bought sriracha by preparing the Do-It-Yourself Sriracha recipe (page 37). Or look for a sugar-free option.

For the sauce

2 tablespoons gluten-free soy sauce

2 tablespoons rice vinegar

1 teaspoon sesame oil

2 garlic cloves, minced

1 tablespoon ginger, minced

¼ teaspoon Do-It-Yourself Sriracha

For the cabbage rolls

2 cups Napa cabbage, finely chopped

1½ teaspoons sea salt

½ pound ground turkey breast

2 tablespoons ginger, minced

4 garlic cloves, finely minced

1 tablespoon sesame oil

1 tablespoon gluten-free soy sauce

1 egg, beaten

4 large Napa cabbage leaves

Nut-free

RELEASE

Dinner

PER SERVING
CALORIES: 200
CARBS: 6G
FAT: 10G
PROTEIN: 20G
SUGAR: 1G

To make the sauce

1. In a small bowl, whisk together the soy sauce, vinegar, sesame oil, garlic, ginger, and sriracha. Set aside. »

Slow Cooker Turkey Cabbage Rolls *continued*

To make the cabbage rolls

1. Put the chopped cabbage in a colander, and sprinkle it with the salt. Let it drain for 20 minutes. The salt will pull the moisture out of the cabbage. After the cabbage has drained, wrap it in a cotton tea towel, and wring out any excess moisture over the sink.

2. In a large bowl, combine the drained cabbage, turkey, ginger, garlic, sesame oil, soy sauce, and beaten egg. Use your hands to mix until well combined.

3. Divide the turkey mixture into four portions, and wrap each in a large cabbage leaf, using a wooden toothpick to secure them, if necessary. Place the cabbage rolls, seam side down, in the bottom of a slow cooker.

4. Pour the sauce over the cabbage rolls and place the cover on the slow cooker. Cook on high for 4 to 5 hours, or on low for 8 to 10 hours.

RELEASE

Dinner

Pork Chops with Mushrooms

SERVES 4 / PREP TIME: 10 MINUTES / COOK TIME: 20 MINUTES

Pork and mushrooms go well together because they both have a slightly sweet, earthy flavor. Use thin-cut, bone-in pork chops. Cooking meat with the bone in adds flavor while it cooks, and the bones can be removed before serving, if you wish.

Ingredient tip: *You can replace the button mushrooms with any in-season mushrooms. Try something different, such as chanterelles or oyster mushrooms, or a blend of wild mushrooms. When cooking mushrooms, the best way to get great flavor from them is to leave them in contact with the pan in a single layer for 6 to 7 minutes before stirring. Then stir them occasionally, cooking until the liquid from the mushrooms has evaporated, another 3 to 4 minutes.*

4 bone-in thin-cut pork chops

½ teaspoon kosher salt, divided

½ teaspoon freshly ground black pepper

2 tablespoons olive oil, divided

2 shallots, minced

8 ounces sliced button mushrooms

½ cup low-sodium vegetable broth

1 tablespoon chopped fresh thyme

2 tablespoons chopped fresh chives

Nut-free

RELEASE

Dinner

PER SERVING
CALORIES: 187
CARBS: 4G
FAT: 10G
PROTEIN: 22G
SUGAR: 1G

1. Sprinkle the pork chops with ¼ teaspoon salt and the pepper.

2. In a large cast iron skillet, heat 1 tablespoon oil over medium-high heat until it shimmers. Working in batches, add the pork chops. Cook, turning once, until the chops cook through, 5 to 7 minutes total. Remove to a platter and tent with foil.

3. Add the remaining 1 tablespoon oil to the pan. Add the shallots and mushrooms. Cook, stirring occasionally, until the mushrooms are browned, about 7 minutes.

4. Add the broth and the remaining ¼ teaspoon salt. Cook, scraping any browned bits from the bottom of the pan, until the liquid is mostly evaporated, 1 to 3 minutes. Stir in the thyme and chives.

5. Serve the pork chops topped with the mushroom sauce.

Slow Cooker Beanless Chili with Peppers and Summer Squash

SERVES 6 / PREP TIME: 15 MINUTES / COOK TIME: 5 TO 10 HOURS IN A SLOW COOKER

Ground turkey and lots of chopped vegetables make this chili low in fat and carbs, and high in protein, fiber, and vitamins. This chili freezes well and will keep in a tightly sealed container in the freezer for up to six months.

2 tablespoons olive oil

1 pound ground turkey breast

1 red onion, chopped

1 green bell pepper, seeded and chopped

1 red bell pepper, seeded and chopped

2 medium zucchini, chopped

1 (14-ounce) can chopped tomatoes, undrained

½ cup water

2 tablespoons chili powder

½ teaspoon ground cumin

Dash of cayenne pepper

Sea salt

Nut-free
Paleo-friendly

RELEASE

Dinner

PER SERVING
CALORIES: 231
CARBS: 10G
FAT: 11G
PROTEIN: 23G
SUGAR: 5G

1. In a large, nonstick sauté pan, heat the olive oil until it shimmers over medium-high heat.

2. Add the turkey and cook, crumbling with a spoon, until it is browned, about 7 minutes.

3. Add the turkey to the slow cooker.

4. Add the onion, green bell pepper, red bell pepper, zucchini, tomatoes, water, chili power, cumin, and cayenne to the slow cooker. Season with salt.

5. Cover and cook on high for 4 to 5 hours, or on low for 8 to 10 hours.

Beef with Broccoli

SERVES 4 / PREP TIME: 10 MINUTES / COOK TIME: 10 MINUTES

Cut the beef into very thin strips so it cooks quickly, and cut it across the grain so it is tender. To thicken the sauce, simmer until it reduces by half.

Serving tip: *You can serve this on cauliflower rice (see Slow Cooker Red Pepper Stuffed with Italian Ground Turkey and Cauliflower, page 160, which explains how to make cauliflower rice), which is low in carbs and fat. Make your own Do-It-Yourself Sriracha (page 37) or look for sugar-free sriracha sauce at your local grocery store.*

5 cups bite-size broccoli florets

1 tablespoon minced garlic

1 tablespoon minced fresh ginger

3 tablespoons gluten-free soy sauce

½ teaspoon salt

12 ounces flank steak

1 tablespoon Do-It-Yourself Sriracha

2 teaspoons sesame oil

2 teaspoons rice wine vinegar

2 tablespoons olive oil, divided

2 scallions, thinly sliced

2 tablespoons sesame seeds

Nut-free

RELEASE

Dinner

PER SERVING
CALORIES: 323
CARBS: 6G
FAT: 21G
PROTEIN: 27G
SUGAR: 1G

1. Place a steamer in a large sauté pan, and add water to a level just below the bottom of the steamer. Bring the water to a boil over high heat. Add the broccoli, cover, and cook for 4 minutes. Remove the broccoli from the steamer and drain.

2. In a large bowl, combine the garlic, ginger, soy sauce, and salt. Add the beef to the mixture and coat well.

3. In a small bowl, mix the sriracha, sesame oil, and rice wine vinegar. Set aside.

4. In a large sauté pan, heat 1 tablespoon olive oil over high heat. Add the beef in a single layer. Cook for 1 minute, stir, and cook for 1 minute more. Transfer to a plate. »

Beef with Broccoli *continued*

5. Add the remaining 1 tablespoon olive oil to the pan. Add the steamed broccoli, and cook for 2 minutes. Stir in the sriracha mixture and cook, stirring frequently, until the liquid reduces by half. Return the beef to the pan, and cook until it is reheated, about 1 minute longer.

6. Serve garnished with the scallions and sesame seeds.

RELEASE

Dinner

Raspberry Sauce

SERVES 12 (2 TABLESPOONS PER SERVING) / PREP TIME: 5 MINUTES

Raspberries are one of the lowest-carbohydrate fruits. Still, you should eat this sauce in moderation during Stage Two to maintain a low-carb, low-fat diet. Serve it with plain, unsweetened almond milk yogurt or coconut milk yogurt.

Ingredient tip: *This sauce freezes well. Portion 2-tablespoon servings into an ice cube tray, then freeze. Melt a cube in a saucepan as you need it.*

1½ cups fresh or frozen raspberries
Juice of 1 lemon
¼ teaspoon powdered stevia
Pinch fine sea salt

1. In a blender, combine the raspberries, lemon juice, stevia, and salt. Blend until the ingredients form a sauce.

2. Strain through a fine-mesh sieve to remove the seeds before serving.

Nut-free
Paleo-friendly
Vegan

RELEASE

Dessert

PER SERVING
CALORIES: 32
CARBS: 8G
FAT: 0G
PROTEIN: 0G
SUGAR: 7G

Lemon Granita

SERVES 8 / PREP TIME: 15 MINUTES, PLUS CHILLING AND FREEZING TIME / COOK TIME: 5 MINUTES

Serve this refreshing lemon granita by itself or with Raspberry Sauce (page 211). For a sweet yet intense lemon flavor, choose Meyer lemons if they are in season.

Ingredient tip: *Agar is a red algae that works as a thickener. You can find it at your local health food store or from online sources. While this recipe calls for powdered stevia, you can replace it with 3 or 4 drops of liquid stevia.*

Nut-free
Paleo-friendly
Vegan

RELEASE

Dessert

PER SERVING
CALORIES: 21
CARBS: 5G
FAT: 0G
PROTEIN: 0G
SUGAR: 0G

1 cup water
½ teaspoon agar powder
½ teaspoon powdered stevia
Strips of lemon zest from 1 lemon
Juice of 3 large lemons

1. In a medium saucepan, heat the water, agar, and stevia over medium-high heat until the stevia and agar are completely dissolved and the water simmers.

2. Stir in the lemon zest strips, remove from the heat, and set aside until the liquid cools. Cover and transfer to the refrigerator to chill completely.

3. Discard the lemon zest. Stir in the lemon juice.

4. Spread the mixture in a thin layer on a baking sheet. Place the sheet in the freezer, and let it freeze completely.

5. Break the lemon mixture into chunks, and place it in the bowl of a food processor. Process until the mixture is smooth but still frozen, or put the chunks in a zip-top plastic bag, and break them up with a hammer.

6. Serve immediately.

Cranberry-Orange Compote

SERVES 4 / PREP TIME: 5 MINUTES / COOK TIME: 25 MINUTES

Cranberries aren't just for the holidays. The berries are very low in carbohydrates, so they make a perfect dessert during this stage of the diet. Orange zest and cinnamon add flavor, while stevia brings just a hint of sweetness. The compote keeps well in the refrigerator, tightly sealed, for up to one week.

4 cups fresh or frozen cranberries

2 cups water

Zest of 1 orange

1 teaspoon ground cinnamon

½ teaspoon powdered stevia

Nut-free
Paleo-friendly
Vegan

RELEASE

Dessert

PER SERVING
CALORIES: 45
CARBS: 12G
FAT: 0G
PROTEIN: 0G
SUGAR: 4G

1. In a large saucepan, heat the cranberries and water over medium-high heat until the cranberries start to pop.

2. Add the orange zest, cinnamon, and stevia.

3. Cook for 15 minutes more to allow the flavors to blend.

4. Serve warm or at room temperature.

Coconut-Chia Pudding

SERVES 4 / PREP TIME: 5 MINUTES, PLUS 3 HOURS TO OVERNIGHT TO CHILL

Chia is high in omega-3 fatty acids and fiber. It also contains calcium, magnesium, and iron. When chia seeds soak in liquid, they turn into a viscous gel that slows the uptake of sugars in your digestive system. When combined with coconut milk, they make a delicious and satisfying low-carb dessert.

⅓ cup chia seeds
1½ cups light coconut milk
1 packet stevia
½ teaspoon vanilla extract

Nut-free
Paleo-friendly
Vegan

RELEASE

Dessert

PER SERVING
CALORIES: 65
CARBS: 4G
FAT: 4G
PROTEIN: 2G
SUGAR: 1G

1. In a small bowl, stir together the chia seeds, coconut milk, stevia, and vanilla.
2. Cover and refrigerate for at least 3 hours or overnight.

Blueberries with Coconut Cream

SERVES 2 / PREP TIME: 10 MINUTES

Coconut cream is made with the solids from coconut milk. It's very easy to make, and it's creamy, delicious, and low in carbs. When combined with low-glycemic-index blueberries, this makes the perfect light and creamy dessert that's high in antioxidants. Don't use light coconut milk for this, or it won't turn out right.

Technique tip: *To make coconut cream, leave a can of full-fat coconut milk in the refrigerator overnight. In the morning, when you open the can, you'll see that a thick layer of cream has settled on top. Spoon the cream from the top of the can, leaving the liquid in the bottom to use for something else.*

4 tablespoons coconut cream

1 packet stevia

½ teaspoon vanilla extract

½ cup blueberries

1. In a small bowl, whisk together the coconut cream, stevia, and vanilla.
2. Divide the blueberries among two bowls.
3. Top with the coconut cream mixture.

Nut-free
Paleo-friendly
Vegan

RELEASE

Dessert

PER SERVING
CALORIES: 120
CARBS: 8G
FAT: 8G
PROTEIN: 1G
SUGAR: 5G

Pumpkin Pie Mousse

SERVES 4 / PREP TIME: 20 MINUTES, PLUS 4 HOURS TO CHILL /
COOK TIME: 5 MINUTES

This mousse relies on gelatin to give it shape and texture. It's low in carbs because it is sweetened with stevia. It's also full of healthy nutrients from the pumpkin, including vitamin A, vitamin B$_6$, vitamin C, and magnesium. Use light coconut milk to keep the fat down. Be sure to choose a puréed pumpkin that doesn't contain any spices, flavorings, or sugar.

Nut-free
Paleo-friendly

RELEASE

Dessert

PER SERVING
CALORIES: 106
CARBS: 10G
FAT: 6G
PROTEIN: 5G
SUGAR: 2G

2 cups light coconut milk, divided

2 tablespoons unflavored gelatin

¼ teaspoon vanilla extract

¼ teaspoon ground cinnamon

¼ teaspoon ground nutmeg

¼ teaspoon ground cloves

Pinch salt

4 packets stevia

1 cup puréed pumpkin

1. In a small bowl, combine 1 cup coconut milk and the gelatin. Stir to combine.

2. In a large saucepan, combine the remaining 1 cup of coconut milk, vanilla, cinnamon, nutmeg, cloves, salt, and stevia, and bring to a simmer. Remove from the heat.

3. Whisk in the reserved coconut milk and gelatin. Whisk until all the gelatin has dissolved.

4. Whisk in the pumpkin purée to combine.

5. Pour into individual dessert dishes, and chill, covered, for at least 4 hours or until the gelatin sets.

Avocado Chocolate Mousse

SERVES 4 / PREP TIME: 10 MINUTES, PLUS CHILL TIME

Here's a good-for-you version of chocolate mousse that tastes delicious and won't make you feel guilty. The avocado, which packs plenty of potassium and heart-healthy fatty acids, gives this dessert richness and a creamy, dense texture.

1 avocado, peeled and pitted

2 tablespoons unsweetened cocoa powder

2 packets stevia

2 tablespoons light coconut milk

½ teaspoon almond extract

Pinch salt

1. In a blender or the bowl of a food processor fitted with a metal chopping blade, process the avocado, cocoa powder, stevia, coconut milk, almond extract, and salt until smooth, about 1 minute.

2. Pour into individual dessert dishes, and chill, covered, until set.

Paleo-friendly
Vegan

RELEASE

Dessert

PER SERVING
CALORIES: 229
CARBS: 12G
FAT: 21G
PROTEIN: 3G
SUGAR: 1G

Hot Chocolate

SERVES 1 / PREP TIME: 5 MINUTES / COOK TIME: 5 MINUTES

Sometimes you just need chocolate. This low-carb, low-fat, sugar-free version is very satisfying. Try it swirled with a cinnamon stick to add extra flavor.

Substitution tip: *If you'd like to add other flavors to your hot chocolate, try flavored stevia drops in any flavor you like in place of the powdered stevia. You can find flavored stevia drops at your local health food store. A little bit of liquid stevia goes a long way, so start with only a few drops and adjust as needed.*

1 cup unsweetened, unflavored coconut milk

3 tablespoons unsweetened cocoa powder

¼ teaspoon powdered stevia

¼ teaspoon freshly grated nutmeg

Nut-free
Paleo-friendly
Vegan

RELEASE

Dessert

PER SERVING
CALORIES: 85
CARBS: 11G
FAT: 7G
PROTEIN: 3G
SUGAR: 1G

1. In a small saucepan, heat the coconut milk, cocoa powder, and stevia over medium heat.

2. Cook, stirring constantly, until the cocoa powder dissolves and the cocoa is hot. Do not let the mixture boil.

3. Serve topped with freshly grated nutmeg.

Chocolate Pudding

SERVES 4 / PREP TIME: 5 MINUTES, PLUS OVERNIGHT TO CHILL /
COOK TIME: 10 MINUTES

Arrowroot powder thickens this pudding and gives it a lovely sheen. Powdered stevia adds sweetness. Serve the pudding chilled in pretty dessert bowls or cups, topped with a few blueberries, sliced strawberries, or raspberries.

Serving tip: *You can make a low-carb, dairy-free whipped topping for your pudding if you like. Place a can of full-fat coconut milk in the refrigerator overnight. When you open the can, you will see that the coconut cream has separated from the liquid. Scoop the cream off the top and discard the liquid. Serve as is or sweeten it with a small amount of stevia. Because the coconut cream is high in fat, limit yourself to only 1 tablespoon.*

2 tablespoons unsweetened cocoa powder

½ tablespoon arrowroot powder

1 cup unsweetened, unflavored coconut milk

½ teaspoon powdered stevia

1 teaspoon vanilla extract

3 tablespoons slivered almonds, toasted

1. In a medium nonstick saucepan, whisk together the cocoa powder and arrowroot powder. Add the coconut milk and stevia, whisking to combine.

2. Place the pan over medium heat, and bring to a simmer; then turn down the heat.

3. Cook, stirring constantly, until the pudding thickens, about 5 minutes. Remove from the heat, and stir in the vanilla.

4. Chill the pudding, covered, overnight.

5. Serve with toasted almonds sprinkled over the top.

**Paleo-friendly
Vegan**

RELEASE

Dessert

PER SERVING
CALORIES: 51
CARBS: 4G
FAT: 4G
PROTEIN: 2G
SUGAR: 1G

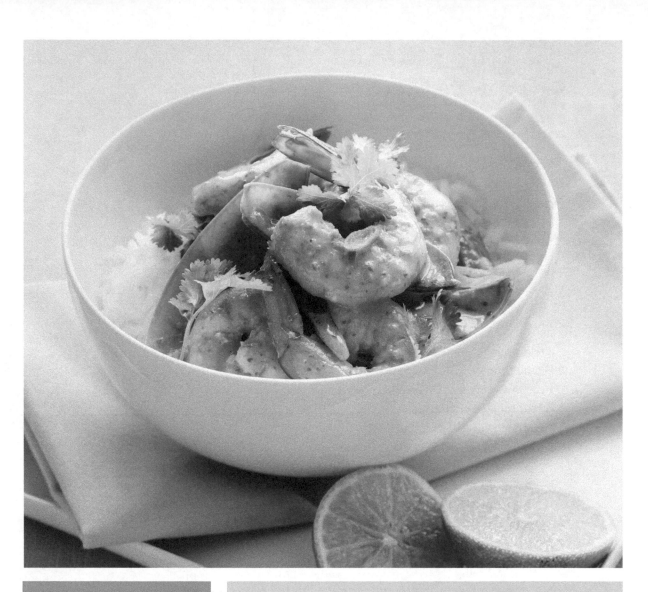

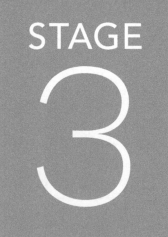

STAGE

3

REIGNITE

STAGE 3 RECIPES

Breakfast

Lunch

Snacks

Dinner

Dessert

Fruit and Greens Smoothie

SERVES 2 / PREP TIME: 5 MINUTES

Prepackaged kale or spinach makes prep for this recipe even faster. If you're using baby kale or spinach, you need not remove the tender stems before use. In Stage Three, rice milk is not an option, because of its high glycemic index. Instead, use unsweetened almond milk, which has a lower glycemic index. You can also use unsweetened coconut milk.

2 tablespoons chia seeds

1 cup unsweetened, unflavored almond milk

3 packed cups chopped fresh kale or spinach leaves

1 cup blueberries

1 small green apple, cored, peeled, and chopped

¼ teaspoon powdered stevia (optional)

1. In a small bowl, stir the chia seeds into the almond milk, and set aside for 10 minutes to allow the chia to thicken.

2. In the bowl of a blender, combine the chia–almond milk mixture, kale, blueberries, apple, and stevia, if using.

3. Blend until all the fruits and vegetables are puréed. Serve immediately.

Paleo-friendly
Vegan

REIGNITE

Breakfast

PER SERVING
CALORIES: 128
CARBS: 25G
FAT: 4G
PROTEIN: 3G
SUGAR: 15G

Steel-Cut Oats with Walnuts and Spices

SERVES 2 / PREP TIME: 5 MINUTES, PLUS OVERNIGHT SOAKING /
COOK TIME: 20 MINUTES

While steel-cut oats contain high levels of carbohydrates, they are reasonably low on the glycemic index, which means your body burns them slowly. Do not replace these oats with quick oats, which have a higher glycemic index that doesn't fit with Stage Three of this plan. Because steel-cut oats take a while to cook, soak them overnight in boiled water, which reduces the cooking time in the morning to just a few minutes.

Time-saving tip: *You can cook this oatmeal in the slow cooker overnight. Put all of the ingredients in the slow cooker except the walnuts, and set it on low before going to bed. In the morning, stir in the walnuts and serve.*

Vegan

REIGNITE

Breakfast

PER SERVING
CALORIES: 374
CARBS: 56G
FAT: 11G
PROTEIN: 14G
SUGAR: 0G

2½ cups water

1 cup steel-cut oats

⅔ cup unsweetened, unflavored almond milk

2 tablespoons coarsely chopped walnuts

¼ teaspoon ground cinnamon

¼ teaspoon ground nutmeg

1. Before going to bed, bring the water to a boil over high heat in a small saucepan. Remove it from the heat. Stir in the oats and cover the pan. Leave it to rest overnight.

2. In the morning, return the pan to the stovetop, and bring it to a boil over high heat. Cook, stirring occasionally, until the oats are tender, about 15 minutes.

3. Stir in the almond milk, walnuts, cinnamon, and nutmeg.

4. Cook until the oats are soft and creamy, about 3 minutes more.

Coconut Yogurt and Berry Parfait with Walnuts

SERVES 2 / PREP TIME: 10 MINUTES / COOK TIME: 5 MINUTES

Berries have a lower glycemic index than many other fruits, and they are packed with antioxidants and phytonutrients. For best results, choose fresh berries. If you can't find coconut yogurt, you can also use cultured almond yogurt. Both are available in many health food stores.

2 tablespoons chopped walnuts

2 cups unsweetened plain cultured coconut yogurt

1 tablespoon honey

½ cup blueberries, divided

½ cup raspberries, divided

Paleo-friendly
Vegetarian

REIGNITE

Breakfast

PER SERVING
CALORIES: 247
CARBS: 40G
FAT: 10G
PROTEIN: 5G
SUGAR: 20G

1. Put the walnuts in a dry sauté pan, and heat them over medium-high heat. Cook, shaking the pan frequently to stir the walnuts, until they are fragrant, about 5 minutes. Remove from the heat, and let the walnuts cool.

2. In a small bowl, whisk together the yogurt and honey.

3. In two parfait glasses, spoon ¼ cup each of the blueberries in the bottom of the glass. Top with ½ cup yogurt.

4. Spoon ¼ cup each of the raspberries on top of the yogurt, and top with ½ cup each of yogurt.

5. Sprinkle the toasted walnuts over the top

Almond Flour Pancakes with Orange-Blueberry Topping

SERVES 4 / PREP TIME: 20 MINUTES / COOK TIME: 15 MINUTES

This recipe replaces white flour with almond meal flour, which you can find at your local natural foods store. Almond flour has a lower glycemic index than white flour, and it contains vitamin E and polyunsaturated fatty acids. The berries add antioxidants, making this a very nutritious, low-glycemic-index breakfast.

Paleo-friendly
Vegetarian

REIGNITE

Breakfast

PER SERVING
CALORIES: 124
CARBS: 13G
FAT: 7G
PROTEIN: 5G
SUGAR: 8G

For the topping

2 cups blueberries

Zest of 1 orange

¼ teaspoon ground cinnamon

1 packet stevia

¼ cup water

For the pancakes

1 cup almond flour

2 eggs, beaten

¼ cup water

Pinch salt

¼ teaspoon ground nutmeg

Coconut oil for cooking

To make the topping

1. In a medium saucepan, combine the blueberries, orange zest, cinnamon, stevia, and water. Bring to a simmer over medium-high heat.

2. Reduce the temperature to medium-low, and simmer, stirring occasionally, until the blueberries soften and turn into a sauce, about 10 minutes.

3. Remove from the heat, and set aside.

To make the pancakes

1. In a small bowl, whisk together the almond flour, eggs, water, salt, and nutmeg until well combined.

2. Heat a griddle or nonstick sauté pan over medium-high heat. Melt about 1 teaspoon of coconut oil on the griddle, and swirl to coat.

3. Drop large spoonfuls of batter onto the hot griddle, and cook until set on one side, about 4 minutes. Flip the pancakes, and cook on the other side until done, about 4 minutes more.

4. Serve with hot blueberry topping.

Scrambled Eggs Florentine

SERVES 4 / PREP TIME: 10 MINUTES / COOK TIME: 15 MINUTES

Spinach and red bell peppers are both filled with healthy antioxidants and fiber, making them very satisfying. Sprinkling pine nuts over the top after cooking adds a healthy dose of omega-3 fatty acids, which are essential to create the proper fatty acid balance in your diet.

Time-saving tip: *To save time, you can use jarred roasted red peppers in place of the red bell pepper. Drain and slice the peppers. Then cook the peppers and spinach together for about 3 minutes before adding the eggs in step 2.*

Paleo-friendly
Vegetarian

REIGNITE

Breakfast

PER SERVING
CALORIES: 206
CARBS: 6G
FAT: 17G
PROTEIN: 9G
SUGAR: 2G

2 tablespoons extra-virgin olive oil

1 medium red bell pepper, seeded and diced

9 ounces baby spinach

1 garlic clove, minced

4 eggs, beaten

¼ teaspoon fine sea salt

¼ teaspoon freshly ground black pepper

Dash of cayenne pepper

¼ cup pine nuts

¼ cup packed, torn fresh basil leaves

1. In a large sauté pan, heat the olive oil over medium-high heat until it shimmers. Add the bell pepper and cook until it softens, about 5 minutes. Add the spinach and cook until it softens and wilts, an additional 3 minutes. Add the garlic and cook until it is fragrant, about 30 seconds. Reduce the heat to medium.

2. While the vegetables cook, in a small bowl whisk together the eggs, salt, pepper, and cayenne.

3. Pour the eggs over the vegetables, and cook, stirring frequently, until the eggs are set, about 3 minutes.

4. Remove the pan from the heat. Stir in the pine nuts and basil, and serve immediately.

Vegetable and Egg Baked Breakfast

SERVES 4 / PREP TIME: 10 MINUTES / COOK TIME: 20 MINUTES

This baked breakfast takes only a few minutes of prep time, but it yields a colorful, delicious, and healthy meal that is filled with nutrients and fiber. The protein will keep you full longer, and the slow-burning carbohydrates will help provide fuel throughout the morning. Substitute any mushrooms you like for the portobellos.

Nonstick cooking spray
3 tablespoons extra-virgin olive oil
Juice of 1 lemon
Zest of ½ lemon
1 large garlic clove, minced
9 ounces fresh baby spinach
2 portobello mushrooms, stems and gills removed, caps cut into ¼-inch slices
1 large beefsteak tomato, sliced
4 eggs
Fine sea salt
Freshly ground black pepper

Nut-free
Paleo-friendly
Vegetarian

REIGNITE

Breakfast

PER SERVING
CALORIES: 189
CARBS: 6G
FAT: 15G
PROTEIN: 9G
SUGAR: 2G

1. Preheat the oven to 400°F.

2. Place an oven rack in the middle of the oven. Lightly spray a 9-by-13-inch baking dish with nonstick cooking spray

3. In a small bowl, whisk together the olive oil, lemon juice, lemon zest, and garlic to make a vinaigrette.

4. In a large bowl, toss the spinach, mushrooms, and tomato slices with the vinaigrette. Arrange the vegetables in the bottom of the baking dish.

5. Make four "nests" in the vegetables. Carefully crack an egg into each nest. Season the eggs with salt and pepper.

6. Bake until the eggs are set and the vegetables soften, 15 to 20 minutes.

Sautéed Cabbage with Poached Eggs

SERVES 2 / PREP TIME: 15 MINUTES / COOK TIME: 15 MINUTES

Sautéed cabbage and onions are a delicious and flavorful base for poached eggs. The cabbage adds fiber and vitamin C as well. If you don't like cabbage, you can replace it with grated zucchini and carrots. (For instructions on poaching an egg, see Summer Squash and Radish Hash with Poached Eggs, page 134.)

Serving tip: *Serve this dish alongside two slices of cooked turkey bacon or a slice of extra-lean Canadian bacon for a balanced and delicious low-glycemic-index breakfast.*

Nut-free
Paleo-friendly
Vegetarian

REIGNITE

Breakfast

PER SERVING
CALORIES: 232
CARBS: 11G
FAT: 19G
PROTEIN: 7G
SUGAR: 5G

2 tablespoons extra-virgin olive oil

2 cups cabbage, shredded

1 onion, thinly sliced

2 garlic cloves, minced

½ teaspoon sea salt

¼ teaspoon freshly ground black pepper

1 tablespoon vinegar

2 eggs

2 tablespoons chopped fresh chives

1. In a large saucepan, heat the olive oil over medium-high heat until it shimmers.

2. Add the cabbage and onion, and cook, stirring occasionally, until the cabbage has softened and is starting to brown, about 12 minutes.

3. Add the garlic and cook, stirring constantly, until it is fragrant, about 30 seconds.

4. Season with salt and pepper, and set aside.

5. In a medium saucepan filled three quarters with water and the vinegar, bring the liquid to a simmer over medium-high heat. Reduce the heat to medium-low, and add the eggs.

6. Poach the eggs until the whites solidify, about 5 minutes.

7. Spoon the cabbage onto two plates. Remove the poached eggs with a slotted spoon, and carefully place atop the cabbage.

8. Garnish with the chopped fresh chives.

Tex-Mex Eggs with Black Beans and Avocados

SERVES 4 / PREP TIME: 10 MINUTES / COOK TIME: 20 MINUTES

This hearty, spicy breakfast takes its cue from traditional huevos rancheros. Avocados add a dose of healthy fats, while black beans have a low glycemic index and a slow burn for sustained energy. Spice it up with a drizzle of your favorite hot sauce.

Ingredient tip: *Liquid smoke adds a hint of smokiness to this breakfast skillet. Be sparing with it, though, because a little goes a very long way.*

2 tablespoons extra-virgin olive oil

1 onion, chopped

1 jalapeño pepper, seeded and chopped

2 garlic cloves, minced

1 (15-ounce) can black beans, rinsed and drained

½ teaspoon chipotle chili powder

Dash of liquid smoke

4 eggs, beaten

¼ cup chopped fresh cilantro

1 avocado, peeled, pitted, and diced

1 large beefsteak tomato, seeded and diced

Hot sauce, for serving

Nut-free
Paleo-friendly
Vegetarian

REIGNITE

Breakfast

PER SERVING
CALORIES: 491
CARBS: 54G
FAT: 22G
PROTEIN: 23G
SUGAR: 4G

1. In a large nonstick sauté pan, heat the olive oil over medium-high heat until it shimmers. Add the onion and jalapeño, and cook, stirring occasionally, until soft, about 5 minutes.

2. Add the garlic and cook, stirring constantly, until the garlic is fragrant, about 30 seconds.

3. Add the black beans, chipotle powder, and liquid smoke. Cook, stirring frequently, until the beans are heated through, about 5 minutes.

4. Add the eggs and cook, stirring frequently, until the eggs are set, about 4 minutes. Remove from the heat.

5. Stir in the cilantro, avocado, and tomato. Serve drizzled with hot sauce.

Softboiled Eggs with Sweet Potato and Apple Hash

SERVES 4 / PREP TIME: 15 MINUTES / COOK TIME: 10 MINUTES

Carefully scoop softboiled eggs out of their shell, and serve them on this delicious sweet and savory fall hash. The result is a satisfying breakfast that is high in vitamin A and fiber. Serve alongside a Turkey Breakfast Sausage patty (page 142) or two slices of turkey bacon for added protein.

Technique tip: *Peeling softboiled eggs can be tricky. However, they are much easier to peel if they have been in the refrigerator for a while. To peel the eggs, plunge them into cold water when they are done cooking. Then, keeping the eggs underwater the whole time, crack each egg on the bottom of the bowl of water. Remove it from the bowl, and peel it under running water.*

Nut-free
Paleo-friendly
Vegetarian

REIGNITE

Breakfast

PER SERVING
CALORIES: 262
CARBS: 29G
FAT: 23G
PROTEIN: 13G
SUGAR: 15G

4 eggs

2 tablespoons extra-virgin olive oil

1 sweet potato, peeled and cut into ¼-inch dice

1 apple, peeled, cored, and cut into ¼-inch dice

½ onion, chopped

½ teaspoon dried sage

2 garlic cloves, minced

½ teaspoon sea salt

¼ teaspoon freshly ground black pepper

1. Fill a large saucepan half full with water, and bring it to a boil over high heat. Reduce the heat to medium, and keep the water at a simmer.

2. Using a spoon or tongs, carefully lower the eggs into the water.

3. Cook for 5 minutes. Remove the eggs from the water, and plunge them into a bowl of cold water.

4. In a large nonstick sauté pan, heat the olive oil over medium-high heat until it shimmers.

5. Add the sweet potato, apple, onion, and sage, and cook, stirring occasionally, until the potatoes soften and brown slightly, about 10 minutes.

6. Add the garlic and cook, stirring constantly, until it is fragrant, about 30 seconds.

7. Season with salt and pepper.

8. Peel the softboiled eggs.

9. Divide the apple mixture between two plates. Carefully split a peeled softboiled egg over each plate of hash to serve.

REIGNITE

Breakfast

Sweet Potato, Pepper, Sausage, and Egg Casserole

SERVES 8 / PREP TIME: 15 MINUTES / COOK TIME: 30 MINUTES

Sweet potato adds a slightly sweet and flavorful component to this easy breakfast casserole. The casserole will keep in the refrigerator for up to five days, so it's a great meal to make on the weekend and warm up for breakfasts all week long.

Substitution tip: *You can replace the sweet potatoes with an equal amount of grated zucchini for a lower-carb version of this casserole.*

Nut-free
Paleo-friendly

REIGNITE

Breakfast

PER SERVING
CALORIES: 257
CARBS: 6G
FAT: 14G
PROTEIN: 25G
SUGAR: 3G

Nonstick cooking spray

2 tablespoons olive oil

1 pound uncooked Turkey Breakfast Sausage (page 142)

1 red bell pepper, chopped

1 onion, chopped

1 garlic clove, minced

12 eggs

1 teaspoon onion powder

1 teaspoon dried sage

½ teaspoon sea salt

¼ teaspoon freshly ground black pepper

1 large sweet potato, peeled and grated

1. Preheat the oven to 375°F. Lightly spray the inside of a 9-inch-square square baking pan with nonstick cooking spray.

2. In a large nonstick sauté pan, heat the olive oil over medium-high heat until it shimmers. Add the turkey sausage and cook, crumbling with a spoon, until it is browned, about 5 minutes.

3. Add the bell pepper and onion, and cook, stirring occasionally, until the vegetables are soft, about 5 minutes more.

4. Add the garlic and cook, stirring constantly, until it is fragrant, about 30 seconds.

5. Remove from the heat and set aside.

6. In a large bowl, whisk together the eggs, onion powder, sage, salt, and pepper.

7. Stir in the sweet potato and cooked turkey sausage mixture, folding to combine.

8. Pour the mixture into the prepared pan. Bake until the casserole sets in the middle, about 30 minutes.

REIGNITE

Breakfast

Canadian Bacon and Bell Pepper Omelet

SERVES 2 / PREP TIME: 5 MINUTES / COOK TIME: 10 MINUTES

Canadian bacon is cut from a different, less fatty part of the pig than regular bacon, but has the same big flavor. Cook the Canadian bacon until it is caramelized and crisp to bring out the sweet, smoky flavors in the meat.

1 tablespoon olive oil

2 slices (1 ounce) Canadian bacon, diced

1 shallot, diced

½ green bell pepper, seeded and cut into ¼-inch pieces

2 eggs

2 egg whites

¼ cup unsweetened, unflavored almond milk

⅛ teaspoon fine sea salt

⅛ teaspoon freshly ground black pepper

Paleo-friendly

REIGNITE

Breakfast

PER SERVING
CALORIES: 200
CARBS: 4G
FAT: 14G
PROTEIN: 16G
SUGAR: 2G

1. In a large sauté pan over medium heat, heat the olive oil until it shimmers. Add the Canadian bacon, shallot, and bell pepper, and cook until the bacon begins to caramelize, about 6 minutes.

2. Meanwhile, in a small bowl, whisk together the eggs, egg whites, almond milk, salt, and pepper.

3. Pour the egg mixture into pan. Reduce the heat to medium-low, and continue cooking until the eggs start to set, about 1 minute.

4. Using a spatula, gently pull the set eggs away from the sides of the pan, and tilt the pan to allow the unset eggs to run into the gaps around the edges. Cook until the eggs set.

5. Fold the omelet over and serve.

Turkey Bacon and Root Vegetable Hash with Poached Eggs

SERVES 2 / PREP TIME: 20 MINUTES / COOK TIME: 15 MINUTES

This hash is wonderful in the fall when farmers' markets are filled with their root vegetable harvest. Cutting the vegetables in ¼-inch dice helps them soften quickly. (For instructions on poaching an egg, see Summer Squash and Radish Hash with Poached Eggs, page 134.)

Ingredient substitution: *Other root vegetables you can use in this hash include celeriac (celery root), sweet potatoes, rutabagas, and parsnips.*

2 tablespoons extra-virgin olive oil

4 slices turkey bacon, chopped into pieces

1 large daikon radish, peeled and cut into ¼-inch dice

2 carrots, peeled and cut into ¼-inch dice

2 turnips, peeled and cut into ¼-inch dice

½ onion, finely chopped

½ teaspoon sea salt

¼ teaspoon freshly ground black pepper

1 teaspoon chopped fresh rosemary

1 tablespoon vinegar

2 eggs, shells removed

Nut-free
Paleo-friendly

REIGNITE

Breakfast

PER SERVING
CALORIES: 304
CARBS: 19G
FAT: 19G
PROTEIN: 14G
SUGAR: 10G

1. In a large sauté pan over medium-high heat, heat the olive oil until it shimmers.

2. Add the turkey bacon, and cook until it begins to brown, about 5 minutes.

3. Add the radish, carrots, turnips, onion, salt, pepper, and rosemary. Cook, stirring occasionally, until the vegetables soften and begin to brown, 7 to 10 minutes.

4. Meanwhile, in a large saucepan filled half full with water and the vinegar, bring the liquid to a simmer over medium-high heat. Reduce the heat to medium-low so the water simmers.

5. Add the eggs to the water, and poach them until the whites solidify, about 5 minutes.

6. Divide the hash between two plates. Top each with a poached egg.

Shrimp Chowder with Fennel

SERVES 6 / PREP TIME: 20 MINUTES / COOK TIME: 25 MINUTES

Most chowders contain dairy products and are thickened with a roux made of flour and fat. This metabolism-boosting chowder is thickened with puréed vegetables instead. The fennel adds a fragrant touch to the shrimp, which is full of beneficial omega-3 fatty acids.

3 tablespoons extra-virgin olive oil, divided

3 slices turkey bacon, chopped into pieces

2 onions, chopped

4 garlic cloves, minced

6 cups low-sodium chicken broth

4 carrots, peeled and chopped

2 stalks celery, chopped

3 white-fleshed sweet potatoes, peeled and cut into ½-inch cubes

1 bulb fennel, diced, fronds reserved

1 pound medium shrimp, peeled and deveined

Sea salt

Freshly ground black pepper

Nut-free
Paleo-friendly

REIGNITE

Lunch

PER SERVING
CALORIES: 312
CARBS: 40G
FAT: 10G
PROTEIN: 15G
SUGAR: 5G

1. In a large pot, heat the olive oil over medium-high heat until it shimmers. Add the turkey bacon and cook, stirring occasionally, until it is crisp, about 5 minutes. Remove the turkey bacon from the fat with a slotted spoon and set aside on a platter.

2. Add the onions to the same pot and cook, stirring occasionally, until they soften, about 5 minutes.

3. Add the garlic and cook, stirring constantly, until fragrant, about 30 seconds.

4. Add the broth to the pot, scraping any browned bits off the bottom.

5. Add the carrots, celery, sweet potatoes, and fennel bulb. Simmer until the vegetables are soft, about 15 to 20 minutes.

6. Using a slotted spoon, transfer about half the cooked vegetables to a blender or a food processor fitted with a metal chopping blade. Try to get as little liquid with the vegetables as possible.

7. Carefully process the vegetables until smooth, about 1 minute, allowing steam to escape through the open top chute of the processor or the vent in the lid of the blender.

8. Use a rubber scraper to scrape the puréed vegetables back into the soup pot. Stir to combine.

9. Return the bacon to the pot, and add the shrimp. Stir to combine.

10. Bring the pot to a simmer and cook, stirring occasionally, for about 5 minutes or until the shrimp turns pink.

11. Add about 2 tablespoons chopped fennel fronds to the soup, and stir to combine. Serve immediately.

REIGNITE

Lunch

Cobb Salad with Shrimp

SERVES 4 / PREP TIME: 15 MINUTES / COOK TIME: 2 MINUTES

Traditional Cobb salad calls for blue cheese dressing. Here, the dressing is dairy-free, so it's lighter and won't slow down your metabolism. The eggs and shrimp offer plenty of protein to help keep you satisfied.

4 tablespoons olive oil, divided

½ teaspoon sweet paprika

½ teaspoon dried oregano

¼ teaspoon dried basil

¼ teaspoon garlic powder

¼ teaspoon celery seed

¼ teaspoon freshly ground black pepper

1 pound uncooked medium shrimp, peeled and deveined

Juice of 1 lime

¼ cup Easy Homemade Mayonnaise (page 37)

1 head romaine lettuce, torn into pieces

1 Roma tomato, cut into ½-inch dice

½ avocado, cut into ½-inch dice

2 hardboiled eggs, cut in quarters

2 slices turkey bacon, cooked and diced

¼ cup minced fresh basil

Nut-free
Paleo-friendly

REIGNITE

Lunch

PER SERVING
CALORIES: 435
CARBS: 8G
FAT: 33G
PROTEIN: 31G
SUGAR: 3G

1. In a small bowl, combine 2 tablespoons olive oil with the paprika, oregano, dried basil, garlic powder, celery seed, and pepper. Add the shrimp, and toss until it is evenly coated.

2. Heat the remaining 2 tablespoons olive oil in a cast iron skillet over medium-high heat. Add the shrimp in a single layer, and cook until they just begin to turn pink, about 1 minute. Turn the shrimp over, and cook until they are cooked through, about 1 minute more. Set aside.

3. In a small bowl, whisk together the lime juice and mayonnaise until smooth.

4. In a large salad bowl, combine the lettuce, tomato, avocado, eggs, and bacon. Toss with the dressing.

5. Add the shrimp and basil, and toss again.

Crab and Artichoke Salad–Stuffed Avocados

SERVES 4 / PREP TIME: 15 MINUTES

Cooked lump crabmeat and canned artichoke hearts taste delicious with creamy avocados. The smoked paprika adds a nice, rich flavor. Choose artichoke hearts packed in water, not marinated hearts. Use the Easy Homemade Mayonnaise (page 37) to dress the salad.

Ingredient tip: *The best way to get lemon zest is to use a rasp-style grater. Use light pressure only, so that you don't remove any of the white pith underneath the flavorful peel. The pith is bitter, so you want to avoid it.*

1 cup cooked lump crabmeat, picked over and rinsed

1 cup water-packed canned artichoke hearts, drained and roughly chopped

3 scallions, minced

4 tablespoons Easy Homemade Mayonnaise

1 lemon, halved

Zest of ½ lemon

¼ teaspoon Do-It-Yourself Sriracha (page 37) or sugar-free sriracha sauce

½ teaspoon smoked paprika

½ teaspoon sea salt

¼ teaspoon freshly ground black pepper

2 Haas avocados, halved lengthwise, pits removed

Nut-free
Paleo-friendly

REIGNITE

Lunch

PER SERVING
CALORIES: 221
CARBS: 14G
FAT: 19G
PROTEIN: 4G
SUGAR: 2G

1. In a medium bowl, combine the crabmeat, artichoke hearts, and scallions. Toss to combine.

2. In a small bowl, whisk together the mayonnaise, juice from half the lemon, lemon zest, sriracha, smoked paprika, salt, and pepper. Pour the dressing over the crab mixture, and stir gently.

3. Using a large spoon, carefully scoop the avocado halves out of the peel, keeping each half intact.

4. Use a spoon to scoop out a little more room in the center for the salad. Reserve any scooped-out avocado for another use.

5. Put the avocados on a plate, and rub the cut, unjuiced lemon half over the surface of the flesh to keep it from turning brown.

6. Scoop the crab salad into the avocado halves. Serve immediately.

Crab Cakes with Sriracha Mayonnaise

SERVES 2 / PREP TIME: 5 MINUTES / COOK TIME: 6 MINUTES

Most commercial crab cakes are made with wheat flour. This recipe calls for flax meal as a binder instead, with the added bonus that it is high in omega-3 fatty acids. To make the flax meal, grind flaxseed in a blender, food processor, or spice grinder until it takes on the consistency of flour.

Substitution tip: *You can replace the crab with flaked halibut for a delicious fish cake.*

½ pound cooked jumbo lump crabmeat, picked over and flaked

1 egg, beaten

½ red bell pepper, minced

4 scallions, minced

¼ cup flax meal

1 teaspoon garlic powder

1 teaspoon Old Bay seasoning

¼ teaspoon fine sea salt

¼ teaspoon freshly ground black pepper

Dash of cayenne pepper

1 teaspoon olive oil

¼ cup Easy Homemade Mayonnaise (page 37)

Juice of ½ lemon

½ teaspoon Do-It-Yourself Sriracha (page 37) or sugar-free sriracha sauce

1. In a medium bowl, combine the crabmeat, egg, bell pepper, scallions, flax meal, garlic powder, Old Bay seasoning, salt, pepper, and cayenne. Stir until the ingredients are just combined. Form the mixture into two patties.

2. In a large sauté pan, heat the olive oil over medium-high heat until it shimmers. Add the crab cakes to the pan, and cook until the cakes are browned, about 3 minutes per side.

3. While the crab cakes cook, in a small bowl whisk together the mayonnaise, lemon juice, and sriracha. Spoon the sriracha mayonnaise over the warm crab cakes, and serve.

Nut-free
Paleo-friendly

REIGNITE

Lunch

PER SERVING
CALORIES: 203
CARBS: 6G
FAT: 20G
PROTEIN: 11G
SUGAR: 1G

Tuna Salad

SERVES 4 / PREP TIME: 15 MINUTES

You don't need mayonnaise to make this delicious classic, but if you can't live without it, use the Easy Homemade Mayonnaise recipe (page 37). Many commercial varieties of mayonnaise contain high-fructose corn syrup or other sweeteners. To flavor the mayonnaise, add a little chopped fresh tarragon if you like.

Substitution tip: *You can replace the tuna in this salad with cooked and diced shrimp or crab. For a little crunch, add some chopped fresh celery or minced fennel.*

2 (6-ounce) cans water-packed albacore tuna, drained and flaked

1 cup canned, drained artichoke hearts, chopped

1 jarred red pepper in oil, drained and cut into ¼-inch pieces

½ cup chopped black olives

Juice of 1 lemon

1½ teaspoons chopped fresh oregano

4 large Bibb (butterhead) lettuce leaves

1 large beefsteak tomato, seeded and chopped

1. In a medium bowl, combine the tuna, artichokes, red pepper, olives, lemon juice, and oregano.

2. Spoon the tuna salad into the lettuce leaves. Top with the chopped tomato.

Nut-free
Paleo-friendly

REIGNITE

Lunch

PER SERVING
CALORIES: 147
CARBS: 7G
FAT: 3G
PROTEIN: 24G
SUGAR: 2G

Chicken Salad with Broccoli and Tomatoes

SERVES 4 / PREP TIME: 15 MINUTES / COOK TIME: 30 MINUTES

The bright cherry tomatoes cheer up this dish. Feel free to swap green beans for the broccoli during the summer and cooked rotisserie chicken (skin and bones removed) in place of the poached chicken when you're in a rush.

2 cups low-sodium chicken broth

2 boneless, skinless chicken breasts

1 carrot, peeled and diced

1 celery rib, diced

2 bay leaves

1 head broccoli, cut into florets

¼ cup olive oil

Juice of 1 lime

1 teaspoon dried oregano

¼ teaspoon fine sea salt

¼ teaspoon freshly ground black pepper

1 pint cherry tomatoes, halved

3 scallions, minced

1. In a large saucepan, bring the broth to a boil over medium-high heat. Add the chicken, carrot, celery, and bay leaves. Cover and simmer gently until the chicken is cooked through, about 20 minutes.

2. Remove the chicken from the poaching liquid, and allow it to cool completely. When cool, cut into ½-inch dice.

3. Place a steamer in a large saucepan, and add water to a level just below the bottom of the steamer. Bring the water to a boil over high heat. Put the broccoli florets in the steamer, cover, and cook until tender, about 8 minutes. Remove the broccoli from the heat, and run it under cold water to stop the cooking. Drain thoroughly, and set aside to cool.

4. In a small bowl, whisk together the olive oil, lime juice, oregano, salt, and pepper to make the vinaigrette.

5. In a large bowl, combine the cooled chicken, broccoli, tomatoes, and scallions. Pour the vinaigrette over the salad, and toss to combine.

Ginger Chicken Slaw

SERVES 4 / PREP TIME: 15 MINUTES

This traditional slaw features two updated twists that make it a wonderful meal. First, it has poached chicken to give the slaw some protein. Second, it uses a ginger-infused dressing to provide a delicious, exotic flavor.

Time-saving tip: *Replace the cabbage, carrots, scallions, and celery with a packaged coleslaw blend to save time. You can find these blends with the bagged salads in the produce section of the grocery store.*

4 ounces boneless, skinless cooked chicken breast, cut into bite-size pieces

4 cups shredded green cabbage

2 carrots, peeled and grated

3 scallions, minced

2 celery ribs, minced

⅓ cup rice wine vinegar

3 tablespoons extra-virgin olive oil

1 tablespoon honey

1 teaspoon Dijon mustard

2 teaspoons grated fresh ginger

Fine sea salt

Freshly ground black pepper

Nut-free
Paleo-friendly

REIGNITE

Lunch

PER SERVING
CALORIES: 213
CARBS: 14G
FAT: 12G
PROTEIN: 11G
SUGAR: 9G

1. In a large bowl, toss together the chicken, cabbage, carrots, scallions, and celery.

2. In a small bowl, whisk together the rice wine vinegar, olive oil, honey, mustard, and ginger. Taste and season the dressing with salt and pepper.

3. Pour the dressing over the vegetables, and toss to coat.

Chicken Caesar Salad with Cashews

SERVES 4 / PREP TIME: 15 MINUTES

In the dressing for this Caesar salad, egg yolk is replaced by toasted cashews, which makes it creamy and thick. If cashews are too sweet for your taste, replace them with sunflower seeds. Anchovy paste adds the classic salty, rich flavor to this updated Caesar. Look for tubes of anchovy paste near the canned tuna at the supermarket.

Substitution tip: *If you don't like anchovies, you can replace the anchovy paste with 1 tablespoon of Worcestershire sauce.*

1½ pounds boneless, skinless cooked chicken breast, cut into 1-inch pieces
12 cups torn romaine lettuce
¼ cup toasted cashews
Juice of 3 lemons
1 garlic clove, minced
1 tablespoon Dijon mustard
1 teaspoon anchovy paste
¼ teaspoon fine sea salt
¼ teaspoon freshly ground black pepper
3 tablespoons olive oil

1. In a large bowl, toss the chicken with the lettuce.
2. In a blender, blend the cashews, lemon juice, garlic, mustard, anchovy paste, salt, and pepper until combined.
3. With the blender running, add the oil in a thin stream through the hole in the lid until the oil is incorporated and the dressing emulsifies.
4. Pour the dressing over the chicken and lettuce, and toss to coat.

Paleo-friendly

REIGNITE

Lunch

PER SERVING
CALORIES: 448
CARBS: 8G
FAT: 23G
PROTEIN: 58G
SUGAR: 2G

Italian Chopped Salad with Ham, Tomatoes, and Peppers

SERVES 4 / PREP TIME: 15 MINUTES

Along with healthy vegetables, this salad has plenty of beneficial fats from the black olives and olive oil. Use lean ham, or even turkey ham, to keep saturated animal fats to a minimum. Red peppers add vitamin C, while artichoke hearts add beneficial fiber, vitamin B$_6$, and magnesium.

1 head iceberg lettuce, cored and chopped

2 plum tomatoes, chopped

1 (14-ounce) can black olives, drained

1 (15-ounce) can water-packed artichoke hearts, drained and chopped

1 red bell pepper, seeded and chopped

4 scallions, chopped

¼ cup basil leaves, torn in pieces

8 ounces lean ham, cubed

2 tablespoons red wine vinegar

¼ cup extra-virgin olive oil

2 garlic cloves, minced

1 tablespoon minced shallots

½ teaspoon Dijon mustard

½ teaspoon sea salt

¼ teaspoon freshly ground black pepper

Nut-free
Paleo-friendly

REIGNITE

Lunch

PER SERVING
CALORIES: 269
CARBS: 16G
FAT: 18G
PROTEIN: 14G
SUGAR: 5G

1. In a large bowl, combine the lettuce, tomatoes, olives, artichoke hearts, bell pepper, scallions, basil, and ham. Toss to combine.

2. In a small bowl, whisk together the red wine vinegar, olive oil, garlic, shallots, mustard, salt, and pepper. Whisk until combined.

3. Pour the dressing over the salad, and toss to coat. Serve immediately.

Ham and Egg Salad Sandwich

SERVES 2 / PREP TIME: 10 MINUTES

These days, many mayonnaise manufacturers use soybean oil, which is cheaper to produce than mayonnaise made with healthier oils such as grapeseed or olive oil. But a diet rich in these oils helps boost "good" cholesterol. If you can find a decent commercially made olive or grapeseed oil mayonnaise that doesn't contain high-fructose corn syrup or sugar, use that. Otherwise, use the Easy Homemade Mayonnaise (page 37).

4 hardboiled eggs

1 tablespoon red wine vinegar

2 tablespoons mayonnaise

2 scallions, minced

4 slices whole-grain gluten-free sandwich bread

4 slices country ham

2 cups baby arugula

1 large beefsteak tomato, sliced

Nut-free

REIGNITE

Lunch

PER SERVING
CALORIES: 439
CARBS: 31G
FAT: 27G
PROTEIN: 20G
SUGAR: 7G

1. In a medium bowl, mash the eggs with a potato masher or fork. Stir in the red wine vinegar, mayonnaise, and scallions.

2. Place a slice of bread on each of two plates. Put two slices of ham on each slice of bread. Place arugula and tomato on the ham. Top with the egg salad.

3. Top each sandwich with another slice of bread and serve.

Turkey Bacon, Lettuce, Tomato, and Avocado Sandwich

SERVES 2 / PREP TIME: 5 MINUTES / COOK TIME: 7 MINUTES

Bacon and tomato are a classically delicious flavor combination. Make this sandwich when tomatoes are in season with fresh, locally grown, organic heirloom tomatoes for an extra flavor boost. The avocado adds a creamy, herbaceous note to this lovely twist on an American classic.

Substitution tip: *To give this sandwich a delicious, peppery bite, replace the lettuce with arugula.*

6 slices turkey bacon

½ avocado

Juice of ½ lemon

½ teaspoon hot sauce

¼ teaspoon sea salt

4 slices whole-grain gluten-free sandwich bread, toasted

4 large slices tomato

2 large pieces lettuce

Nut-free

REIGNITE

Lunch

PER SERVING
CALORIES: 337
CARBS: 44G
FAT: 15G
PROTEIN: 16G
SUGAR: 2G

1. In a large, nonstick sauté pan, cook the turkey bacon over medium-high heat until it is brown and crispy, about 7 minutes. Drain the bacon on paper towels and set aside.

2. In a small bowl, using a fork, mash together the avocado, lemon juice, hot sauce, and salt.

3. Spread the avocado mixture on two of the pieces of toast.

4. Lay 3 slices of bacon on top of the avocado spread on each sandwich. Top with 2 tomato slices and a lettuce slice.

5. Top each sandwich with another slice of bread and serve.

Slow Cooker Sloppy Joe Lettuce Cups with Avocado Slaw

SERVES 6 / PREP TIME: 20 MINUTES / COOK TIME: 4 TO 10 HOURS IN A SLOW COOKER

Instead of serving sloppy Joes on high-carbohydrate buns made from white flour, scoop it into large pieces of lettuce and eat it with a fork. The avocado and cabbage slaw adds a satisfying crunch, while the sloppy Joe mixture itself is packed with delicious vegetables.

Substitution tip: *Instead of lettuce cups, serve the sloppy Joes on large grilled portobello mushroom caps.*

**Nut-free
Paleo-friendly**

REIGNITE

Lunch

PER SERVING
CALORIES: 365
CARBS: 27G
FAT: 17G
PROTEIN: 27G
SUGAR: 16G

For the sloppy Joes

2 tablespoons olive oil

1 pound ground turkey breast

1 onion, chopped

1 green bell pepper, seeded and chopped

1 red bell pepper, seeded and chopped

1 medium zucchini, chopped

2 (14-ounce) cans crushed tomatoes

2 tablespoons apple cider vinegar

2 tablespoons pure maple syrup

1 tablespoon Dijon mustard

½ teaspoon sea salt

½ teaspoon freshly ground black pepper

6 large iceberg lettuce leaves

For the slaw

2 cups shredded cabbage

2 carrots, peeled and grated

3 scallions, chopped

1 avocado, peeled and pitted

3 tablespoons apple cider vinegar

2 garlic cloves, minced

¼ teaspoon sea salt

¼ teaspoon freshly ground black pepper

To make the sloppy Joes

1. In a large, nonstick sauté pan, heat the olive oil over medium-high heat until it shimmers. Add the ground turkey and cook, crumbling with a spoon, until it is browned, 5 to 7 minutes. Put the turkey in the slow cooker.

2. Add the onion, green bell pepper, red bell pepper, zucchini, tomatoes, apple cider vinegar, maple syrup, mustard, salt, and pepper to the slow cooker.

3. Cover and cook on high for 4 to 5 hours, or on low for 8 to 10 hours.

4. When it's time to serve, spoon the sloppy Joe mix into the lettuce leaves, and top with the slaw.

To make the slaw

1. In a medium bowl, combine the cabbage, carrots, and scallions. Toss to mix.

2. In a blender, blend the avocado, apple cider vinegar, garlic, salt, and pepper until smooth.

3. Pour the avocado mixture over the cabbage mixture, and toss to combine.

REIGNITE

Lunch

Fruit and Fennel Yogurt

SERVES 4 / PREP TIME: 5 MINUTES / COOK TIME: 5 MINUTES

Rhubarb is naturally quite tart, but a little bit of stevia takes away the bite. Fennel is a natural partner for the rhubarb. Do not cook the rhubarb more than about four minutes, or it will turn to mush.

Ingredient tip: *You can find coconut yogurt at your local health food store—it might be labeled "cultured coconut milk." You can replace coconut yogurt with almond yogurt. Always choose plain, unsweetened yogurt.*

¼ cup water

½ teaspoon powdered stevia

3 cups thinly sliced fresh rhubarb

1 cup thinly sliced fennel

1½ cups sliced strawberries

1 cup plain unsweetened coconut yogurt

Nut-free
Vegan

REIGNITE

Snacks

PER SERVING
CALORIES: 68
CARBS: 13G
FAT: 5G
PROTEIN: 1G
SUGAR: 4G

1. In a medium saucepan, bring the water and stevia to a boil over medium-high heat. Add the rhubarb and cook, stirring occasionally, until the rhubarb is just beginning to soften, 3 to 4 minutes.

2. Remove the pan from the heat, and transfer the rhubarb to a large bowl to cool.

3. Stir the sliced fennel and strawberries into the cooled rhubarb mixture. Serve it spooned over coconut yogurt.

Cannellini Bean Salad with Mint

SERVES 4 / PREP TIME: 15 MINUTES

While this recipe calls for cannellini beans, you can use any white bean. White beans have a neutral flavor that allows the fresh herbs and other ingredients to shine. The beans also add fiber and protein to this salad.

Substitution tip: *You can add any vegetables you like to this salad. Consider sliced red bell pepper or chopped cool cucumbers for crunch and additional interesting flavors.*

2 (15-ounce) cans cannellini beans, rinsed and drained

2 (15-ounce) can artichoke hearts, drained and halved

12 cherry tomatoes, halved

½ red onion, minced

¼ cup olive oil

1 tablespoon red wine vinegar

¼ cup finely chopped fresh mint

¼ cup finely chopped fresh flat-leaf parsley

1 garlic clove, minced

1 tablespoon minced shallot

⅛ teaspoon red pepper flakes

Fine sea salt

Freshly ground black pepper

**Nut-free
Vegan**

REIGNITE

Snacks

PER SERVING
CALORIES: 413
CARBS: 60G
FAT: 14G
PROTEIN: 21G
SUGAR: 11G

1. In a large bowl, combine the cannellini beans, artichoke hearts, tomatoes, and onion. Toss to combine.

2. In a small bowl, whisk together the olive oil, red wine vinegar, mint, parsley, garlic, shallot, and red pepper flakes.

3. Pour the vinaigrette over the bean mixture, and toss to combine. Season with salt and pepper.

Crispy Baked Spiced Chickpeas

SERVES 8 / PREP TIME: 5 MINUTES / COOK TIME: 35 MINUTES

Chickpeas, also known as garbanzo beans, are a delicious low-glycemic-index food. When you roast them, they become crispy, making them a delicious and addictive finger food. Dry the chickpeas as thoroughly as possible before cooking them to ensure crispiness and reduce baking time.

½ teaspoon sea salt

½ teaspoon freshly ground black pepper

½ teaspoon white pepper

⅛ teaspoon cayenne pepper

¼ teaspoon smoked paprika

¼ teaspoon garlic powder

¼ teaspoon onion powder

1 (15-ounce) can chickpeas, drained

2 tablespoons olive oil

Nut-free
Vegan

REIGNITE

Snacks

PER SERVING
CALORIES: 93
CARBS: 33G
FAT: 7G
PROTEIN: 10G
SUGAR: 6G

1. Preheat the oven to 400°F. Line a large rimmed baking sheet with parchment paper.

2. In a small bowl, mix the salt, black pepper, white pepper, cayenne, paprika, garlic powder, and onion powder until well blended.

3. In a colander, rinse the chickpeas and thoroughly drain them. Put the chickpeas on several layers of paper towels, and gently pat them dry with another paper towel to absorb as much moisture as possible.

4. In a large bowl, combine the chickpeas, olive oil, and spice mixture. Toss to coat the chickpeas with the oil and spices.

5. Spread the chickpeas in a single layer on the prepared baking sheet. Bake until the chickpeas are crispy and browned, about 35 minutes.

6. Cool before serving.

Spicy Apple Chips

SERVES 2 / PREP TIME: 10 MINUTES / COOK TIME: 2 TO 3 HOURS

These simple apple chips don't take much work. Just slice them thinly, sprinkle on some spices, and leave them to bake in a low-heat oven. Typically, thin chips take about 2 hours to start to crisp. If the chips are thicker, you may need to check on them every 15 minutes or so after that until the apples have reached the desired level of crispiness.

1 apple, core removed, sliced crosswise into ⅛-inch rounds
½ teaspoon ground cinnamon
¼ teaspoon ground ginger
¼ teaspoon ground nutmeg

1. Preheat the oven to 275°F. Line a baking sheet with parchment paper.

2. Place the apples in a single layer on the baking sheet.

3. In a small bowl, mix together the cinnamon, ginger, and nutmeg. Sprinkle the mixture over the apples.

4. Bake for 1 hour. Using a spatula, flip the apples and continue baking for 1 hour more. Check for doneness every 15 minutes after that. The apples are done when they are crisp.

5. Cool on a wire rack before serving.

Nut-free
Paleo-friendly
Vegan

REIGNITE

Snacks

PER SERVING
CALORIES: 51
CARBS: 13G
FAT: 0G
PROTEIN: 0G
SUGAR: 10G

Spiced Pecans

SERVES 12 / PREP TIME: 5 MINUTES / COOK TIME: 10 MINUTES

The secret of these spicy pecans is Chinese five-spice powder, which you can find in the spice section of your grocery store. The powder has a delicious combination of savory and sweet spices that makes these nuts extremely enticing. As a bonus, pecans are high in healthy omega-3 fatty acids.

2 cups pecan halves
2 tablespoons extra-virgin olive oil
2 tablespoons Chinese five-spice powder

1. Preheat the oven to 400°F. Line a rimmed baking sheet with parchment paper.

2. In a medium bowl, toss the pecan halves, olive oil, and Chinese five-spice powder to combine.

3. Spread the nuts on the baking sheet in a single layer. Roast until fragrant, 8 to 10 minutes.

4. Store, tightly sealed, at room temperature for up to 1 week.

Paleo-friendly
Vegan

REIGNITE

Snacks

PER SERVING
CALORIES: 251
CARBS: 5G
FAT: 25G
PROTEIN: 4G
SUGAR: 1G

Red Pepper Hummus with Crudités

SERVES 4 / PREP TIME: 20 MINUTES

Roasted red bell peppers and smoked paprika add a sweet smokiness to this delicious hummus. If you'd like an even smokier flavor, you can roast a sweet red bell pepper on the grill or under the broiler and use it to replace the jarred pepper (see technique tip).

Technique tip: *To roast a pepper, cut it into quarters and remove the seeds. Place the pepper directly on the grill, skin-side down (or under the broiler, skin side up), and grill until the flesh chars, about 12 minutes. Flip the pepper and cook until the flesh is soft, another 10 minutes. Peel off the charred skin, and use as directed in the recipe.*

1 (15-ounce) can chickpeas, rinsed and drained

1 jarred roasted red bell pepper, drained

2 tablespoons olive oil

Juice of 1 lemon

⅓ cup tahini

¼ cup chopped fresh flat-leaf parsley

2 garlic cloves, coarsely chopped

½ teaspoon smoked paprika

¼ teaspoon red pepper flakes

¼ teaspoon ground cumin

¼ teaspoon freshly ground black pepper

12 baby carrots

12 cherry tomatoes

1 large jicama, peeled and cut into 12 sticks

6 celery ribs, halved crosswise

1. In a food processor or blender, combine the chickpeas, roasted red bell pepper, olive oil, lemon juice, tahini, parsley, garlic, paprika, red pepper flakes, cumin, and black pepper.

2. Process until the hummus is smooth, about 2 minutes.

3. Serve with the carrots, tomatoes, jicama, and celery.

Nut-free
Paleo-friendly
Vegan

REIGNITE

Snacks

PER SERVING
CALORIES: 509
CARBS: 67G
FAT: 22G
PROTEIN: 18G
SUGAR: 17G

Root Vegetables with Zesty Black Bean Dip

SERVES 6 / PREP TIME: 15 MINUTES

This spicy dip comes together quickly. Use canned black beans that have been well drained to make the dip. You can serve this with any root vegetables, although this recipe calls for carrots and jicama. Adjust the heat of the dip by adding more or less cayenne. The amount called for in the recipe will make the dip mildly spicy.

1 (15-ounce) can black beans, rinsed and drained

2 tablespoons chopped cilantro

2 tablespoons prepared salsa or pico de gallo (see Breakfast Tacos, page 151)

1 teaspoon ground cumin

¼ teaspoon cayenne pepper

½ teaspoon sea salt

½ red onion, diced

Juice of 1 lime

1 jicama, peeled and sliced

4 carrots, peeled and cut into sticks

1. In a blender of a food processor fitted with a metal chopping blade, combine the black beans, cilantro, salsa, cumin, cayenne, and salt.

2. Process until smooth, about 1 minute. Scrape into a medium bowl.

3. Stir the onion and lime juice into the bean dip.

4. Serve the bean dip with the jicama and carrots for dipping.

Nut-free
Vegan

REIGNITE

Snacks

PER SERVING
CALORIES: 286
CARBS: 55G
FAT: 1G
PROTEIN: 15G
SUGAR: 6G

Roasted Eggplant Spread

SERVES 4 / PREP TIME: 10 MINUTES / COOK TIME: 20 MINUTES

Also known as baba ghanoush, this roasted eggplant dip is delicious the day you make it, but it also improves with time. Make the dip and store it, tightly sealed, in the refrigerator for a day or two to allow the flavors to develop. Serve the dip with wheat-free crackers or cut vegetables.

Substitution tip: *This recipe calls for traditional Italian eggplant. If you'd like, you can substitute the smaller Japanese eggplants. Instead of cutting the smaller eggplants into quarters, halve them and cook them just as you would the Italian eggplant.*

1 large eggplant, quartered lengthwise
2 tablespoons olive oil
3 garlic cloves, minced
¼ cup tahini
Juice of 2 lemons
½ teaspoon freshly grated lemon zest
⅛ teaspoon red pepper flakes
Fine sea salt
Freshly ground black pepper

Nut-free
Vegan

REIGNITE

Snacks

PER SERVING
CALORIES: 181
CARBS: 11G
FAT: 15G
PROTEIN: 4G
SUGAR: 4G

1. Preheat the broiler and adjust the rack to the middle of the oven. Line a baking sheet with parchment paper.

2. Brush the eggplant quarters with the olive oil, and put them on the baking sheet. Put the eggplant under the broiler and cook, turning occasionally, until the eggplant pieces are charred and soft, about 20 minutes. Remove them from the oven, and set aside to cool.

3. When the eggplant is cool, remove the flesh from the skin. Discard the skin.

4. Put the eggplant flesh in a bowl and mash it with a fork.

5. Add the garlic, tahini, lemon juice, lemon zest, and red pepper flakes. Continue mashing and stirring until the dip is well combined.

6. Season with salt and pepper.

Mushroom and Walnut Paté with Pepperoncini and Radish

SERVES 6 / PREP TIME: 20 MINUTES, PLUS 2 HOURS TO CHILL / COOK TIME: 15 MINUTES

While this recipe calls for crimini mushrooms, you can use any variety you find available. Make a canapé from the paté by serving it on a radish round with a pepperoncini pepper slice on top.

½ cup chopped walnuts

4 tablespoons extra-virgin olive oil, divided

16 ounces crimini mushrooms, stems removed, cut into quarters

2 shallots, minced

3 garlic cloves, minced

1 teaspoon fresh thyme, chopped

2 tablespoons Worcestershire sauce

1 tablespoon Dijon mustard

½ teaspoon freshly ground black pepper

2 small daikon radishes, sliced

½ cup sliced rings of pepperoncini peppers

Paleo-friendly

REIGNITE

Snacks

PER SERVING
CALORIES: 180
CARBS: 8G
FAT: 16G
PROTEIN: 5G
SUGAR: 3G

1. In a large sauté pan over medium-high heat, heat the walnuts, shaking the pan back and forth to stir them, until the walnuts are fragrant, about 5 minutes. Remove the walnuts from the heat, and set them aside.

2. In the same pan, heat 2 tablespoons olive oil over medium-high heat until it shimmers. Add the mushrooms and shallots, and cook, stirring occasionally, until the mushrooms are soft and browned, about 7 minutes.

3. Add the garlic and cook, stirring until fragrant, about 30 seconds.

4. In a blender or the bowl of a food processor fitted with a metal chopping blade, combine the mushroom mixture, walnuts, the remaining 2 tablespoons olive oil, thyme, Worcestershire sauce, mustard, and pepper.

5. Process for about 20 one-second pulses, until the mushrooms are nearly smooth. Some texture will remain. Chill the mixture for 2 hours.

6. Spread each radish slice with the mushroom mixture. Top with a pepperoncini ring.

Avocado Deviled Eggs

SERVES 12 / PREP TIME: 15 MINUTES

Avocados replace mayonnaise in these deviled eggs, giving them healthy fats and an interesting green color. Avocados also add fiber, vitamin C, vitamin B₆, and vitamin A to the healthy protein from the eggs. Finish with a sprinkle of smoked paprika to add color and a subtle, surprising flavor.

Time-saving tip: *Many grocery stores now sell hardboiled eggs in the egg section of the store.*

12 hardboiled eggs, peeled and halved lengthwise
1 soft avocado, peeled, pitted, and cut into cubes
Juice of 1 lime
2 scallions, finely minced
½ teaspoon sea salt
1 tablespoon Dijon mustard
Smoked paprika

1. Put the eggs, cut side up, on a platter. Using a spoon, carefully scoop out the yolks and put them in a medium bowl.

2. Add the avocado, lime juice, scallions, salt, and mustard to the yolks.

3. Gently mash the mixture with a fork until it has the consistency of guacamole.

4. Spoon the egg and avocado mixture back into the egg white halves.

5. Sprinkle with smoked paprika.

Nut-free
Paleo-friendly
Vegetarian

REIGNITE

Snacks

PER SERVING
CALORIES: 99
CARBS: 2G
FAT: 8G
PROTEIN: 6G
SUGAR: 0G

Shrimp Ceviche with Avocado

SERVES 4 / PREP TIME: 10 MINUTES, PLUS 6 TO 7 HOURS TO CHILL / COOK TIME: 0 MINUTES

Ceviche, featuring fresh and delicious seafood, comes from coastal Central and South America. While the seafood in ceviche is "cooked," the cooking does not occur via heat. Instead, the acid in the citrus juice cooks the seafood as it chills. The acid also imparts surprising flavors that combine with jalapeño pepper, tomato, and creamy avocado for a delicious snack or appetizer.

Substitution tip: *While this recipe calls for very fresh shrimp, you can also use fresh scallops. Avoid using frozen (or frozen and thawed) shrimp if at all possible. If the thought of not using heat to cook bothers you, you can substitute cooked shrimp or scallops for raw.*

Nut-free
Paleo-friendly

REIGNITE

Snacks

PER SERVING
CALORIES: 143
CARBS: 6G
FAT: 6G
PROTEIN: 14G
SUGAR: 4G

Juice of 2 lemons

Juice of 2 limes

Juice of 1 orange

⅓ cup cilantro, finely chopped

1 medium garlic clove, pressed through a garlic press

1 teaspoon jalapeño pepper, seeded and finely minced

½ pound raw fresh shrimp, peeled, deveined, and cut into small pieces

1 heirloom tomato, seeded and diced

½ avocado, pitted, peeled, and cubed

Sea salt

Freshly ground black pepper

1. In a small bowl, whisk together the lemon juice, lime juice, orange juice, cilantro, garlic, and jalapeño pepper.

2. In a medium bowl, combine the shrimp and tomato. Pour the citrus juice mixture over the top.

3. Cover the bowl, and refrigerate for 6 to 7 hours, allowing the citrus juice to cook the shrimp.

4. Stir in the avocado cubes, and season with salt and pepper just before serving.

Salmon Salad and Zucchini Canapés

SERVES 6 / PREP TIME: 10 MINUTES

Salmon is full of healthy omega-3 fatty acids. It also contains protein. When you combine this healthy smoked salmon in a creamy salad and serve it atop a zucchini round, you have the perfect flavorful and nutritious snack or hors d'oeuvre.

4 tablespoons Easy Homemade Mayonnaise (page 37)

Juice and zest of 1 lemon

2 tablespoons chopped fresh dill, plus sprigs for garnish

¼ teaspoon sea salt

¼ teaspoon freshly ground black pepper

10 ounces smoked salmon, cut into pieces

1 celery stalk, minced

2 tablespoons capers

1 medium zucchini, sliced into rounds

12 cherry tomatoes, halved

1. In a small bowl, whisk together the mayonnaise, lemon juice, lemon zest, chopped dill, salt, and pepper. Set aside.

2. In a medium bowl, mix the salmon, celery, and capers.

3. Add the mayonnaise mixture, and fold to carefully coat the salmon with the dressing.

4. Spoon the salmon salad onto the zucchini rounds. Top with a sprig of fresh dill and a cherry tomato half.

Nut-free

REIGNITE

Snacks

PER SERVING
CALORIES: 147
CARBS: 14G
FAT: 6G
PROTEIN: 12G
SUGAR: 8G

Cantaloupe and Prosciutto

SERVES 2 / PREP TIME: 5 MINUTES

Prosciutto is a cured ham native to northern Italy. Its salty character makes a nice contrast with the fresh fruit. Use 2 cups of cantaloupe for this recipe, and then use the rest for the Cantaloupe Seed Drink (page 120).

2 cups cantaloupe chunks
Juice of 1 lemon
4 slices prosciutto

1. Toss the cantaloupe with lemon juice.
2. Divide the cantaloupe chunks between two plates.
3. Drape two pieces of prosciutto over each plate of cantaloupe, and serve.

Nut-free
Paleo-friendly

REIGNITE

Snacks

PER SERVING
CALORIES: 201
CARBS: 19G
FAT: 5G
PROTEIN: 20G
SUGAR: 18G

Edamame Spinach Salad

SERVES 4 / PREP TIME: 10 MINUTES / COOK TIME: 5 MINUTES

Edamame, or soybeans, are sold frozen and fresh. Buying them already shelled saves one step in preparation. Cool the edamame completely before adding them to the salad.

10 ounces frozen shelled edamame, thawed

1 (15-ounce) can kidney beans, rinsed and drained

1 cup blueberries

½ cup slivered almonds

2 carrots, peeled and cut into ¼-inch rounds

10 ounces baby spinach

10 cherry tomatoes, halved

½ cup olive oil

Juice of 2 lemons

¼ teaspoon fine sea salt

¼ teaspoon freshly ground black pepper

Vegan

REIGNITE

Dinner

PER SERVING
CALORIES: 578
CARBS: 49G
FAT: 36G
PROTEIN: 23G
SUGAR: 15G

1. Fill a large saucepan with water, and bring it to a boil over high heat. Add the edamame, cover, and cook until tender, about 5 minutes. Drain the edamame, and allow them to cool completely.

2. In a large bowl, combine the cooled edamame, kidney beans, blueberries, silvered almonds, carrots, spinach, and tomatoes. Toss to combine.

3. In a small bowl, whisk together the olive oil, lemon juice, salt, and pepper.

4. Pour the dressing over the salad, and toss to coat.

Carrot-Ginger Soup with Kale Pesto

SERVES 6 / PREP TIME: 10 MINUTES / COOK TIME: 30 MINUTES

Carrots have a low glycemic index, so the carbs in this soup will burn slowly. Adding a pesto made with kale, cilantro, and walnuts raises the level of healthy omega-3 fatty acids and adds a lot of flavor to the soup. If you prefer, you can use pine nuts in place of the walnuts, and extra-virgin olive oil in place of the walnut oil.

Technique tip: *When puréeing the soup in the blender, place a folded towel between your hand and the blender lid, and hold the lid firmly in place. After about 10 seconds, carefully remove the cap from the blender lid to let the steam escape through the hole. Replace the cap and blend until smooth, allowing the steam to escape every few seconds.*

Paleo-friendly
Vegan

REIGNITE

Dinner

PER SERVING
CALORIES: 264
CARBS: 23G
FAT: 17G
PROTEIN: 8G
SUGAR: 7G

2 cups chopped fresh kale leaves

½ cup chopped fresh cilantro

¼ cup coarsely chopped walnuts

¼ cup walnut oil

2 tablespoons olive oil

2 tablespoons minced fresh ginger

1 medium onion, chopped

2 garlic cloves, minced

5 cups low-sodium vegetable broth

1 pound carrots, peeled and cut into ¼-inch dice

1. In a food processor or blender, combine the kale, cilantro, walnuts, and walnut oil. Process for 20 to 30 seconds to finely chop the nuts and vegetables, and combine all ingredients. Set the pesto aside.

2. In a large soup pot, heat the olive oil over medium-high heat until it shimmers. Add the ginger and onion and cook, stirring frequently, until the onion is soft and starting to brown, about 7 minutes.

3. Add the garlic and cook, stirring constantly, until fragrant, about 30 seconds.

4. Add the broth and carrots. Cover and cook until the carrots are tender, about 20 minutes.

5. Working in batches if needed, blend the hot soup on high to purée, 20 to 30 seconds.

6. Serve the soup with the pesto spooned on top.

Three-Bean Chili

SERVES 6 / PREP TIME: 15 MINUTES / COOK TIME: 30 MINUTES

Chili is the perfect food for an autumn or winter evening. Beans have a low glycemic index, so the carbs burn slowly, keeping you satisfied. You can use any type of beans you like in this flavorful chili.

Ingredient tip: *If you can't find dried chipotle chili powder in the spice aisle, you can make your own by purchasing dried chipotle chilies and processing them in the food processor or a spice grinder. You can also substitute 1 chopped canned chipotle chili in adobo sauce.*

2 tablespoons olive oil

1 onion, chopped

1 green bell pepper, seeded and chopped

1 red bell pepper, seeded and chopped

1 jalapeño pepper, seeded and chopped

3 garlic cloves, minced

1 (15-ounce) can black beans, rinsed and drained

1 (15-ounce) can kidney beans, rinsed and drained

1 (15-ounce) can pinto beans, rinsed and drained

2 (15-ounce) cans crushed tomatoes, undrained

2 tablespoons chili powder

1 teaspoon chipotle chili powder

1 teaspoon dried oregano

½ teaspoon ground cumin

½ teaspoon fine sea salt

½ teaspoon freshly ground black pepper

¼ teaspoon cayenne pepper

6 scallions, sliced

¼ cup chopped fresh cilantro

Nut-free
Vegan

REIGNITE

Dinner

PER SERVING
CALORIES: 318
CARBS: 51G
FAT: 7G
PROTEIN: 17G
SUGAR: 11G

1. In a large pot, heat the olive oil over medium-high heat until it shimmers. Add the onion, green bell pepper, red bell pepper, and jalapeño. Cook, stirring occasionally, until the vegetables soften and begin to brown, about 6 minutes. »

Three-Bean Chili *continued*

2. Add the garlic and cook, stirring constantly, until it is fragrant, about 30 seconds.

3. Add the black beans, kidney beans, pinto beans, tomatoes and juice, chili powder, chipotle powder, oregano, cumin, salt, black pepper, and cayenne.

4. Reduce the heat to medium, and simmer, stirring frequently, until the flavors blend and the beans are heated through, about 20 minutes.

5. Serve topped with the scallions and chopped fresh cilantro.

REIGNITE

Dinner

Black Bean Burger Wraps

SERVES 4 / PREP TIME: 15 MINUTES / COOK TIME: 20 MINUTES

Black beans hold these bean burgers together—although any type of cooked legumes, such as lentils, black-eyed peas, pinto beans, or adzuki beans, will do. Meanwhile, the mushrooms add a deep, savory flavor, and the aromatic spices give the burgers a delicious Southwest flavor.

4 tablespoons olive oil, divided

6 medium crimini mushrooms, stemmed and sliced

½ onion, chopped

1 jalapeño pepper, seeded and minced

2 garlic cloves, minced

1 teaspoon chipotle chili powder

¼ teaspoon ground cumin

1 (15-ounce) can black beans, rinsed and drained

¼ cup chopped fresh cilantro

Juice of 1 lime

½ teaspoon fine sea salt

¼ teaspoon red pepper flakes

4 large green lettuce leaves

1 avocado, peeled, pitted, and sliced

1 large beefsteak tomato, chopped

Nut-free
Vegan

REIGNITE

Dinner

PER SERVING
CALORIES: 240
CARBS: 18G
FAT: 17G
PROTEIN: 6G
SUGAR: 2G

1. In a large sauté pan, heat 2 tablespoons olive oil over medium-high heat until it shimmers. Add the mushrooms, onion, and jalapeño, and cook until the vegetables are soft, 5 to 7 minutes.

2. Add the garlic cloves, chipotle powder, and cumin. Cook, stirring constantly, until the garlic and spices are fragrant, about 30 seconds. Remove from the heat and set aside.

3. In a large bowl, mash the black beans. Stir in the mushroom mixture, cilantro, lime juice, salt, and red pepper flakes until well combined. Form the mixture into four patties. »

Black Bean Burger Wraps *continued*

4. In a sauté pan, heat the remaining 2 tablespoons olive oil over medium-high heat until it shimmers. Add the bean patties and cook, without moving them, until they brown, about 6 minutes per side.

5. Put each patty on a large lettuce leaf, and top with the avocado and tomato. Wrap the lettuce around the patty to eat.

REIGNITE

Dinner

Brussels Sprout Hash with Eggs and Avocados

SERVES 2 / PREP TIME: 10 MINUTES / COOK TIME: 20 MINUTES

Adding vinegar and red pepper flakes balances the bitter flavor of the Brussels sprouts with heat and acidity, while avocado adds healthy omega-3 fats and a creamy, satisfying texture. The recipe also calls for a touch of stevia for a hint of sweetness to balance the full flavor profile. Prepare the Do-It-Yourself Sriracha recipe (page 37) in advance. Or if you are short on time, look for sugar-free sriracha sauce at your local grocery store.

Time-saving tip: *Thinly slicing the dense Brussels sprouts helps them cook quickly.*

3 tablespoons olive oil, divided

1 onion, cut into thin half moons

1 pound Brussels sprouts, sliced thinly

3 garlic cloves, minced

¼ cup apple cider vinegar

¼ teaspoon Do-It-Yourself Sriracha

Pinch of powdered stevia

Fine sea salt

Freshly ground black pepper

2 eggs

½ avocado, cut into ¼-inch dice

Nut-free
Vegetarian

REIGNITE

Dinner

PER SERVING
CALORIES: 501
CARBS: 36G
FAT: 37G
PROTEIN: 16G
SUGAR: 10G

1. In a large sauté pan, heat 2 tablespoons olive oil over medium-high heat until it shimmers. Add the onion and Brussels sprouts, and cook, stirring occasionally, until the vegetables are soft and beginning to brown, 7 to 8 minutes.

2. Add the garlic and cook until fragrant, about 30 seconds.

3. Add the apple cider vinegar, sriracha, and stevia. Reduce the heat to medium, and simmer, stirring occasionally, until the liquid reduces by half, about 4 minutes. Season with salt and pepper.

4. While the hash cooks, in a medium nonstick sauté pan, heat the remaining 1 tablespoon olive oil over medium heat until the oil shimmers. Carefully crack the eggs into the pan, keeping them separate. Season the eggs with salt and pepper. »

Brussels Sprout Hash with Eggs and Avocados *continued*

5. Cook the eggs until the whites set, about 3 minutes. Carefully flip the eggs, and cook them for another 30 seconds to 1 minute more for over easy, or 2 to 3 minutes for over medium.

6. Divide the hash between two plates. Top each plate of hash with an egg, and then scatter the avocado over all.

REIGNITE

Dinner

Crab and Cauliflower Pilaf

SERVES 4 / PREP TIME: 20 MINUTES / COOK TIME: 5 MINUTES

All varieties of rice have a fairly high glycemic load, so this pilaf recipe replaces rice with a popular low-carb staple, cauliflower. Cauliflower "rice" has a mild flavor, but it holds a nice, rice-like texture that makes it an excellent substitute. To make cauliflower rice, see the recipe for Slow Cooker Red Pepper Stuffed with Italian Ground Turkey and Cauliflower (page 160).

Ingredient tip: You can store cauliflower rice sealed in freezer bags. When you're ready to use the rice, place it on a baking sheet in a single layer and bake at 425°F for 20 minutes, turning occasionally. Use as you would cooked rice in recipes.

2 tablespoons olive oil

1 large leek, cut into ¼-inch rounds, rings separated

1 tablespoon Dijon mustard

¼ teaspoon fine sea salt

¼ teaspoon freshly ground black pepper

3 cups low-sodium vegetable broth

1½ cups cauliflower "rice" (from about 1 small head cauliflower)

1 pound sugar snap peas, trimmed

2 carrots, peeled and julienned

8 ounces cooked lump crabmeat, picked over and flaked

¼ cup pine nuts

2 tablespoons minced fresh tarragon

2 tablespoons minced fresh dill

1 lemon, cut into 6 wedges

Paleo-friendly

REIGNITE

Dinner

PER SERVING
CALORIES: 343
CARBS: 23G
FAT: 20G
PROTEIN: 21G
SUGAR: 9G

1. In a large Dutch oven, heat the olive oil over medium-high heat until it shimmers.

2. Add the leek and cook, stirring frequently, until softened, 3 to 4 minutes.

3. Stir in the mustard, salt, and pepper. Add the broth and stir again, scraping any brown bits from the bottom of the pan. Remove from the heat.

4. Stir in the cauliflower rice, snap peas, carrots, and crabmeat. Cover and allow the mixture to rest until all ingredients warm through, about 5 minutes.

5. Sprinkle with the pine nuts, tarragon, and dill. Serve with lemon wedges.

Mexican Scallops and Mushrooms with Avocado

SERVES 4 / PREP TIME: 10 MINUTES / COOK TIME: 25 MINUTES

Chipotle chile powder gives this dish a subtle heat, while the lime adds acidity for balance. If you can't find chipotle chile powder, grind a whole chipotle chile into powder using a spice grinder or a food processor. You can also substitute chili powder for the chipotle chile powder, although it will lack the smokiness of the chipotle.

Nut-free
Paleo-friendly

REIGNITE

Dinner

PER SERVING
CALORIES: 301
CARBS: 15G
FAT: 18G
PROTEIN: 22G
SUGAR: 4G

2 tablespoons extra-virgin olive oil, divided

1 pound bay scallops

Sea salt

Freshly ground black pepper

½ pound button mushrooms, quartered

1 onion, minced

1 carrot, peeled and julienned

2 garlic cloves, minced

Juice of 2 limes

½ teaspoon chipotle chile powder

1 avocado, peeled, pitted, and cut into ½-inch dice

1. In a large sauté pan, heat 1 tablespoon olive oil over medium-high heat until it shimmers.

2. Season the scallops with salt and pepper. Add them to the hot oil, and cook, stirring occasionally, until they are opaque, 5 to 7 minutes.

3. Remove the scallops from the pan with a slotted spoon, and set them aside on a platter.

4. Add the remaining 1 tablespoon olive oil to the pan, and add the mushrooms. Cook, stirring occasionally, until the mushrooms release their liquid and start to brown, about 7 minutes.

5. Add the onion and carrot to the mushrooms, and cook, stirring frequently, until the vegetables soften, about 5 minutes.

6. Add the garlic to the pan and cook, stirring constantly, until it is fragrant, about 30 seconds.

7. Add the lime juice, chipotle chile powder, and reserved scallops. Cook, stirring constantly, until the scallops heat through, about 3 minutes.

8. Mix the scallop mixture with the avocado, and serve immediately.

Shrimp with Summer Squash

SERVES 4 / PREP TIME: 15 MINUTES / COOK TIME: 15 MINUTES

Any summer squash will work in this recipe. If you're cooking it at the peak of summertime, chances are there's plenty of zucchini or yellow squash available. Use fresh herbs for a bright, fresh summertime flavor. To chiffonade basil, roll several leaves into a roll and then cut the roll crosswise into thin ribbons.

Ingredient tip: *Fresh herbs will keep for a week or longer if you store them appropriately. To store the herbs, make sure they don't have any moisture on the leaves. Then snip off the bottoms of the stems, and put the herbs in a glass of water. For very fresh herbs, try growing a window or planter box of herbs in a sunny location.*

3 tablespoons gluten-free soy sauce

3 teaspoons rice wine vinegar

2 to 3 teaspoons hot sauce

2 tablespoons olive oil

1 small zucchini, diced

4 yellow summer squash, cut into ½-inch dice

2 pounds large shrimp, peeled and deveined

6 scallions, chopped

1 garlic clove, minced

3 tablespoons minced fresh ginger

2 tablespoons minced fresh chives

2 tablespoons fresh basil chiffonade

¼ cup pine nuts, toasted

1. In a small bowl, stir together the soy sauce, rice wine vinegar, and hot sauce until smooth, and set aside.

2. In a nonstick skillet, heat the olive oil over medium-high heat. Add the zucchini and summer squash, and cook, stirring frequently, until the vegetables are just beginning to caramelize, about 5 minutes.

3. Add the shrimp, and cook until it turns pink and the vegetables are tender, about 2 minutes. Add the scallions, garlic, and ginger, and cook until fragrant, about 30 seconds.

4. Stir the soy sauce mixture again, and add it to the skillet. Bring it to a boil, and cook until the liquid reduces slightly, about 2 minutes.

5. Sprinkle with the chives, basil, and pine nuts, and serve.

REIGNITE

Dinner

Calamari Salad

SERVES 4 / PREP TIME: 20 MINUTES / COOK TIME: 1 MINUTE

Calamari, or squid, goes well with the bright acidic flavors in this dressing, as well as the crispiness of the vegetables. If you'd like a slightly different take on this salad, you can replace the celery with chopped fennel and the celery leaves with chopped fennel fronds.

Time-saving tip: *For this tasty salad, ask your fishmonger to slice the calamari into rings for you, or you can buy frozen calamari rings. Completely thaw the frozen calamari quickly by placing it in a zip-top bag and submerging the bag in cold water. Change the water every 30 minutes to keep it cold.*

Nut-free
Paleo-friendly

REIGNITE

Dinner

PER SERVING
CALORIES: 290
CARBS: 12G
FAT: 26G
PROTEIN: 4G
SUGAR: 3G

1½ pounds calamari rings

Juice of 1 lemon

1 tablespoon red wine vinegar

⅓ cup extra-virgin olive oil

1 large garlic clove, minced

½ teaspoon fine sea salt

¼ teaspoon freshly ground black pepper

1 small red onion, chopped

1 cup halved cherry tomatoes

2 celery ribs, cut into ¼-inch pieces, leaves left whole

2 tablespoons finely chopped fresh flat-leaf parsley

1. Fill a large saucepan with water. Bring the water to a boil over high heat. Cook the calamari until it is opaque, 40 to 60 seconds.

2. Drain and immediately transfer to a bowl of ice water to stop the cooking. Drain and pat dry.

3. In a large bowl, whisk together the lemon juice, red wine vinegar, olive oil, garlic, salt, and pepper. Stir in the onion, and let stand for 5 minutes.

4. Add the calamari, tomatoes, celery pieces and leaves, and parsley to the bowl. Toss.

5. Let the salad stand for at least 15 minutes to allow the flavors to develop before serving.

Baked Cod with Tomatoes, Asparagus, and Olives

SERVES 4 / PREP TIME: 10 MINUTES / COOK TIME: 15 MINUTES

This dish works just as well with olives from a can or jar as with fancy olives. There is plenty of salt in the olives, so you probably won't need to season the dish. Taste it before serving, and adjust the seasonings as necessary.

Technique tip: *Choose thin, tender asparagus for this dish. To trim the asparagus, hold it at each end and bend the spear using gentle pressure. It will break at the point where the asparagus grows tough. Discard the tough bottom ends of the asparagus.*

Nut-free
Paleo-friendly

REIGNITE

Dinner

PER SERVING
CALORIES: 390
CARBS: 11G
FAT: 23G
PROTEIN: 32G
SUGAR: 4G

- 5 tablespoons olive oil, divided
- 1½ pounds cod fillets, cut into 4 portions
- ½ teaspoon freshly ground black pepper
- 1 bunch asparagus
- 1 pint cherry tomatoes
- ¼ cup pitted black olives
- ¼ cup green pimiento-stuffed olives
- ¼ cup pepperoncini peppers, stemmed
- ¼ cup diced red onion
- 1 tablespoon red wine vinegar
- ½ teaspoon minced fresh oregano
- ½ teaspoon minced fresh thyme
- 1 teaspoon sesame seeds

1. Preheat the oven to 475°F. Lightly coat a large baking pan with 1 tablespoon olive oil.

2. Place the cod fillets in the prepared pan. Brush the cod with 1 tablespoon olive oil. Season with the black pepper. Bake for 5 minutes.

3. Add the asparagus and tomatoes to the pan, and drizzle with 2 tablespoons olive oil. Return the pan to the oven.

4. Bake until the cod flakes easily when tested with a fork, 7 to 10 minutes. »

Baked Cod with Tomatoes, Asparagus, and Olives *continued*

5. Meanwhile, in a medium bowl combine the black olives, green olives, pepperoncini peppers, onion, the remaining 1 tablespoon olive oil, the red wine vinegar, oregano, thyme, and sesame seeds.

6. Serve the olives spooned over the cooked fish and vegetables.

Macadamia-Crusted Halibut

SERVES 4 / PREP TIME: 15 MINUTES / COOK TIME: 15 MINUTES

You don't need flour or cornstarch to make a tasty coating for fish. This crust also works beautifully for baked chicken. Macadamia nuts add crunch and immense flavor to this mild fish.

Ingredient tip: *Macadamia nuts contain a lot of oil and turn rancid quickly. Buy only as much as you need for the recipe.*

1 egg white

1 tablespoon Dijon mustard

2 tablespoons arrowroot powder

¼ cup crushed toasted macadamia nuts

1 tablespoon chopped fresh oregano

1 tablespoon chopped fresh basil

Zest of 1 lemon

¼ teaspoon fine sea salt

¼ teaspoon freshly ground black pepper

1¼ pounds halibut fillets, cut into 4 portions

4 lemon wedges

Paleo-friendly

REIGNITE

Dinner

PER SERVING
CALORIES: 289
CARBS: 7G
FAT: 11G
PROTEIN: 40G
SUGAR: 1G

1. Preheat the oven to 400°F. Line a rimmed baking sheet with parchment paper.

2. In a shallow dish, whisk together the egg white and mustard.

3. In another shallow dish, put the arrowroot powder.

4. In a third shallow dish, combine the macadamia nuts, oregano, basil, lemon zest, salt, and pepper.

5. Dip each piece of fish in the arrowroot powder, then in the egg mixture, and then in the nut mixture. Place each coated fillet on the prepared baking sheet.

6. Bake until lightly browned on the outside and opaque in the center, 12 to 15 minutes. Serve with lemon wedges.

Salmon with Fennel and Tomato Salad

SERVES 4 / PREP TIME: 15 MINUTES / COOK TIME: 10 MINUTES

Tomato and fennel make a beautiful pairing with this salmon dish. Salmon is high in healthy omega-3 fatty acids, much of which is concentrated in the skin. The skin is not too fatty for Stage Three of this diet, so if you like eating the crispy salmon skin, go ahead and enjoy.

Ingredient tip: *Fennel is in season from late summer until late fall. It has a light licorice flavor and a satisfying crunch that works well with seafood. While most recipes call for the fennel bulb, you can also use fennel fronds as a fresh herb seasoning. To preserve their delicate flavor, add the fronds at the very end of cooking.*

Nut-free
Paleo-friendly

REIGNITE

Dinner

PER SERVING
CALORIES: 340
CARBS: 11G
FAT: 22G
PROTEIN: 29G
SUGAR: 3G

Juice of 3 lemons

3 tablespoons extra-virgin olive oil, divided

¾ teaspoon salt, divided

2 tablespoons chopped fresh tarragon

1 large fennel bulb, cored, halved, and sliced as thinly as possible, fronds minced

1¼ pounds salmon fillet with skin, cut into 4 portions

½ teaspoon ground coriander

¼ teaspoon freshly ground black pepper

2 cups halved cherry tomatoes

2 teaspoons minced fresh chives

1. In a large bowl, whisk together the lemon juice, 2 tablespoons olive oil, ½ teaspoon salt, and the tarragon. Add the fennel slices to the bowl and set aside.

2. Season the salmon with the remaining ¼ teaspoon of the salt, the coriander, and the pepper.

3. In a cast iron skillet, heat the remaining 1 tablespoon oil over medium-high heat until it shimmers. Add the salmon, skin-side down, and cook for 2 minutes. Carefully turn the salmon over, and continue cooking until just opaque in the center, about 4 minutes.

4. Add the tomatoes to the fennel mixture, and toss to combine. Top with the chives and minced fennel fronds. Serve the salad with the salmon.

Horseradish-Crusted Salmon with Baked Asparagus

SERVES 2 / PREP TIME: 5 MINUTES / COOK TIME: 12 MINUTES

This simple salmon dish is packed with flavor, courtesy of the horseradish, which complements the oily and earthy sweetness of salmon. When you add a side of baked asparagus, you have a quick and delicious low-carb meal.

For the asparagus

¾ pound asparagus, woody ends snapped off

2 tablespoons olive oil

Zest of 1 lemon

½ teaspoon sea salt

½ teaspoon freshly ground black pepper

For the salmon

12 ounces salmon fillet

Sea salt

Freshly ground black pepper

1 tablespoon Dijon mustard

2 tablespoons prepared horseradish

2 tablespoons olive oil

Nut-free
Paleo-friendly

REIGNITE

Dinner

PER SERVING
CALORIES: 395
CARBS: 9G
FAT: 40G
PROTEIN: 37G
SUGAR: 5G

To make the asparagus

1. Preheat the oven to 400°F. Line a rimmed baking pan with parchment paper.

2. In a medium bowl, toss the asparagus with olive oil, lemon zest, salt, and pepper.

3. Spread the asparagus in a single layer on the prepared baking pan. Roast until tender, 10 to 12 minutes.

4. Remove the asparagus from the oven and set aside.

To make the salmon

1. Turn the oven to broil.

2. Season the salmon with salt and pepper. »

Horseradish-Crusted Salmon with Baked Asparagus *continued*

3. In a small bowl, whisk together the mustard and horseradish. Set aside.

4. In a large, ovenproof sauté pan, heat the olive oil over medium-high heat until it shimmers.

5. Add the salmon and cook until it browns slightly, about 2 minutes on each side.

6. Spread the mustard and horseradish mixture over the flesh side of the salmon.

7. Transfer the salmon to the broiler, skin side down. Broil until the horseradish mixture forms a crust, 3 to 4 minutes.

8. Serve with a side of asparagus.

REIGNITE

Dinner

Curried Shrimp

SERVES 4 / PREP TIME: 10 MINUTES / COOK TIME: 10 MINUTES

Most recipes call for a bit of sugar to tame the heat of the curry, but you won't miss the sugar in this version. Any curry paste will work for this dish, including yellow or vindaloo. Look for dry-packed scallops, because these haven't been treated with preservatives.

Ingredient note: *Kaffir lime leaves add fragrance to many Thai recipes. They are thick, shiny leaves with a distinct flavor and scent. You can find them at Asian grocery stores. Some markets may also have them in the Asian foods aisle.*

2 tablespoons olive oil

½ onion, sliced

1 fresh red chili pepper, seeded and thinly sliced

1½ tablespoons red curry paste

¾ cup full-fat coconut milk

¼ cup water

1 kaffir lime leaf, cut into ribbons, or the zest of 1 lime

8 ounces medium shrimp, peeled and deveined

¼ teaspoon fish sauce

4 lime wedges

Nut-free
Paleo-friendly

REIGNITE

Dinner

PER SERVING
CALORIES: 301
CARBS: 8G
FAT: 21G
PROTEIN: 23G
SUGAR: 3G

1. In a Dutch oven, heat the olive oil over medium-high heat until it shimmers. Add the onion and chili pepper, and cook, stirring frequently, until the vegetables are soft, about 4 minutes.

2. Add the curry paste, and sauté until it is aromatic, about 1 minute. Add the coconut milk, water, and lime leaf, and bring the curry to a low boil.

3. Add the shrimp to the pot, and cook gently until they are cooked, 1 to 2 minutes. Remove from the heat.

4. Add the fish sauce, and stir just to combine. Serve with lime wedges.

Chef's Salad

SERVES 4 / PREP TIME: 10 MINUTES

This chef's salad uses homemade mayonnaise for its dressing. It's also chock-full of healthy vegetables and delicious lean meats. Top it with crunchy sunflower seeds for a healthy dose of omega-3 fatty acids.

¼ cup Easy Homemade Mayonnaise (page 37)

Juice of 1 lemon

2 tablespoons red wine vinegar

1 garlic clove, minced

1 tablespoon finely minced shallot

1 tablespoon minced fresh chives

¼ teaspoon fine sea salt

¼ teaspoon freshly ground black pepper

2 heads romaine lettuce

1 large beefsteak tomato, chopped

1 red bell pepper, chopped

4 scallions, chopped

4 ounces deli ham, cut into pieces

4 ounces deli turkey, cut into pieces

4 hardboiled eggs, chopped

¼ cup sunflower seeds

Nut-free

REIGNITE

Dinner

PER SERVING
CALORIES: 298
CARBS: 15G
FAT: 20G
PROTEIN: 17G
SUGAR: 8G

1. In a medium bowl, whisk together the mayonnaise, lemon juice, red wine vinegar, garlic, shallot, chives, salt, and pepper.

2. In a large bowl, combine the lettuce, tomato, bell pepper, scallions, ham, turkey, hardboiled eggs, and sunflower seeds. Toss together.

3. Serve the salad with the dressing on the side.

Turkey Meatloaf Muffins

SERVES 4 / PREP TIME: 10 MINUTES / COOK TIME: 30 MINUTES

While most meatloaf has added breadcrumbs, this recipe uses healthy vegetables instead. The vegetables add nutrition, while the ground turkey adds protein. Baking the meatloaf in muffin cups instead of a loaf pan means it cooks quickly—so you can have your dinner ready sooner.

2 tablespoons extra-virgin olive oil

1 onion, chopped

3 garlic cloves, minced

1 pound ground turkey breast

1 egg, lightly beaten

3 carrots, grated

2 cups frozen spinach, pressed, drained, and chopped

2 tablespoons Dijon mustard

1 tablespoon horseradish

1 tablespoon Worcestershire sauce

1 teaspoon dried thyme

1 teaspoon sea salt

½ teaspoon freshly ground black pepper

1. Preheat the oven to 375°F.
2. In a large nonstick sauté pan, heat the olive oil over medium-high heat until it shimmers.
3. Add the onion and cook, stirring occasionally, until it is soft, about 5 minutes.
4. Add the garlic and cook, stirring constantly, until it is fragrant, about 30 seconds.
5. Remove the onion and garlic from the heat, and let them cool.
6. In a large bowl, combine the ground turkey, cooked garlic and onions, egg, carrots, spinach, mustard, horseradish, Worcestershire sauce, thyme, salt, and pepper. Use your hands to mix well.
7. Spoon the mixture into 12 muffin tins.
8. Bake until the meat is cooked through, about 25 minutes.

Nut-free
Paleo-friendly

REIGNITE

Dinner

PER SERVING
CALORIES: 349
CARBS: 10G
FAT: 17G
PROTEIN: 26G
SUGAR: 5G

Chicken Satay with Peanut Sauce

SERVES 4 / PREP TIME: 15 MINUTES, PLUS 2 HOURS TO MARINATE /
COOK TIME: 10 MINUTES

In a restaurant, you usually see chicken satay threaded on wooden skewers. That's handy for grilling, but it isn't necessary if you bake the chicken in the oven. This dish has a big flavor, so all you really need with it is a simple salad.

Ingredient tip: *Most commercial brands of peanut butter contain added sugar and salt. Look for the natural brands, and then read the labels carefully. You want a brand that is sugar-free and unsalted. Natural peanut butter contains no additional oils (which give commercial peanut butter a smooth consistency), but it is often loaded with saturated and trans fats. In natural peanut butter, the peanut oil will separate and rise to the top. Simply stir it in before using. Keeping the peanut butter in the refrigerator will help prevent separation.*

REIGNITE

Dinner

PER SERVING
CALORIES: 224
CARBS: 7G
FAT: 13G
PROTEIN: 22G
SUGAR: 3G

2 tablespoons fish sauce

Juice of 4 limes

1 tablespoon gluten-free soy sauce

1 tablespoon grated fresh ginger

4 garlic cloves, finely minced

Dash of cayenne pepper

12 ounces chicken breast tenders, cut into 1-inch strips

¼ cup smooth peanut butter

¼ cup light coconut milk

Juice of ½ lime

½ teaspoon Do-It-Yourself Sriracha (page 37) or sugar-free sriracha sauce

1. In a medium bowl, whisk together the fish sauce, lime juice, soy sauce, ginger, garlic, and cayenne. Add the chicken and toss to coat.

2. Cover and marinate the chicken in the refrigerator for 2 hours.

3. Preheat the oven to 375°F. Line a rimmed baking sheet with parchment paper.

4. Spread the chicken strips on the pan in a single layer, and bake until fully cooked, about 10 minutes.

5. While the chicken cooks, put the peanut butter, coconut milk, lime juice, and sriracha in a blender or food processor. Process until the sauce is completely combined, about 20 seconds.

6. Serve the chicken with the peanut sauce for dipping.

Pecan-Crusted Chicken Tenders

SERVES 4 / PREP TIME: 10 MINUTES / COOK TIME: 20 MINUTES

There's no need to give up crispy coated chicken. Instead of using flour or breading to make the tenders crisp, coat them in crunchy crushed pecans. The pecans add fiber and healthy essential fatty acids. Serve the chicken tenders with a simple side salad for a complete, healthy meal.

1 cup chopped pecans

1 teaspoon garlic powder

½ teaspoon sea salt

¼ teaspoon freshly ground black pepper

Dash of cayenne pepper

1 egg, beaten

2 tablespoons Dijon mustard

1 pound chicken breast tenders

Paleo-friendly

REIGNITE

Dinner

PER SERVING
CALORIES: 405
CARBS: 5G
FAT: 26G
PROTEIN: 41G
SUGAR: 1G

1. Preheat the oven to 425°F. Line a rimmed baking sheet with parchment paper.

2. In the bowl of a food processor fitted with a metal chopping blade, pulse the pecans, garlic powder, salt, pepper, and cayenne until the pecans are in very small pieces, about 10 one-second pulses. Pour the mixture onto a plate. If you don't have a food processor, chop the pecans with a knife until they form crumbs. Then stir in the garlic powder, salt, pepper, and cayenne.

3. In a small bowl, combine the egg and mustard, and whisk well.

4. Dip each tender in the egg mixture and then in the pecan mixture, coating the entire piece.

5. Put the chicken pieces on the prepared baking sheet. Bake for about 10 minutes, and then turn the chicken over. Continue baking for another 5 to 10 minutes, until the chicken is cooked through.

6. Remove chicken pieces from the oven and serve immediately. You can refrigerate any leftovers and reheat in a toaster oven for another meal.

Chicken Sausage and Hearts of Palm Salad

SERVES 4 / PREP TIME: 10 MINUTES

Use cooked Italian chicken or turkey sausage for this recipe. If you can't find pre-cooked chicken sausage, bake uncooked sausage in a 375° oven for 30 minutes. Allow the sausage to cool completely before slicing and putting it in the salad.

Substitution tip: *If you prefer, you can replace the hearts of palm with water-packed artichoke hearts. Rinse the artichoke hearts, and halve them before using in the salad.*

¼ cup olive oil

3 tablespoons white wine vinegar

2 teaspoons Dijon mustard

½ teaspoon dried tarragon

½ teaspoon dried marjoram

1 teaspoon dried parsley

3 cups cooked Italian-seasoned chicken sausage, cut into 1-inch rounds

1 (14-ounce) can hearts of palm, drained and cut into ½-inch pieces

6 radishes, cut into thin rounds

2 celery ribs, cut into ¼-inch pieces

1 pint cherry tomatoes, halved

1 head butter lettuce, separated into leaves

Nut-free
Paleo-friendly

REIGNITE

Dinner

PER SERVING
CALORIES: 315
CARBS: 12G
FAT: 22G
PROTEIN: 22G
SUGAR: 5G

1. In a small bowl, whisk together the olive oil, white wine vinegar, mustard, tarragon, marjoram, and parsley.

2. In a large bowl, combine the cooked sausage, hearts of palm, radishes, celery, tomatoes, and butter lettuce leaves. Toss together.

3. Pour the dressing over the salad, and toss again before serving.

Veal Piccata

SERVES 4 / PREP TIME: 10 MINUTES / COOK TIME: 10 MINUTES

Veal piccata is a traditional Italian dish that cooks up in a single pan. To make it, use very thin veal scaloppini, which cooks very quickly. Then spoon the piquant lemon-caper sauce over the top.

Substitution tip: *If you don't want to use veal, you can substitute chicken breasts or slices of pork tenderloin.*

Paleo-friendly

REIGNITE

Dinner

PER SERVING
CALORIES: 382
CARBS: 2G
FAT: 26G
PROTEIN: 36G
SUGAR: 1G

2 tablespoons olive oil

4 (4-ounce) veal cutlets, pounded to ¼-inch thickness

Fine sea salt

Freshly ground black pepper

Juice of 2 lemons

¼ cup low-sodium chicken broth

2 tablespoons capers, rinsed

2 tablespoons chopped fresh flat-leaf parsley

¼ cup pine nuts

1. In a large sauté pan, heat the olive oil over medium high heat until it shimmers.

2. Season the veal liberally with salt and pepper.

3. Working in batches, add the veal to the pan and cook until it is cooked through, about 3 minutes per side. Remove the veal from the pan, and set it aside on a platter.

4. Add the lemon juice and broth to the same pan. Scrape any browned bits off the bottom of the pan. Add the capers. Simmer until the liquid reduces to ¼ cup. Remove from the heat. Stir in the parsley and pine nuts.

5. Return the veal to the pan. Turn to coat it in the sauce. Serve the veal with the sauce spooned over the top.

Bison Burgers with Bistro Burger Sauce

SERVES 4 / PREP TIME: 10 MINUTES / COOK TIME: 15 MINUTES

Fish sauce and garlic pump up the savory flavor of these ground bison burgers. Because bison is pastured and not raised on factory farms, the meat is lower in fat and higher in omega-3 fatty acids than ground beef. Therefore, bison cooks more quickly, so you need to watch to make sure it doesn't overcook or burn.

Substitution tip: *You may replace the bison in these burgers with extra-lean grass-fed ground beef or ground turkey breast. If you can't find in-season heirloom tomatoes, substitute a beefsteak or hothouse tomato.*

For the Bistro Burger Sauce

1 egg yolk

1 tablespoon red wine vinegar

¼ teaspoon fine sea salt

¾ cup olive oil

1 tablespoon Worcestershire sauce

1 tablespoon gluten-free soy sauce

1 garlic clove, finely minced

½ teaspoon pure maple syrup

2 tablespoons chopped fresh chives

For the burgers

1 pound ground bison

1 teaspoon fish sauce

1 garlic clove, minced

1 teaspoon freshly ground black pepper

1 teaspoon smoked paprika

½ teaspoon fine sea salt

Pinch of powdered stevia

2 tablespoons olive oil

4 gluten-free hamburger buns

4 tablespoons Bistro Burger Sauce

1 large heirloom tomato, sliced

1 bunch arugula »

Nut-free

REIGNITE

Dinner

PER SERVING
CALORIES: 533
CARBS: 37G
FAT: 29G
PROTEIN: 33G
SUGAR: 5G

Bison Burgers with Bistro Burger Sauce *continued*

To make the Bistro Burger Sauce

1. In a blender or food processor, combine the egg yolk, red wine vinegar, and salt.

2. With the blender or food processor running, add the olive oil one drop at a time through the top. After about 10 drops of oil, add the oil in a very thin stream until it is completely incorporated.

3. Scrape the mixture into a small bowl. Stir in the Worcestershire sauce, soy sauce, garlic, maple syrup, and chives.

To make the burgers

1. In a large bowl, combine the ground bison, fish sauce, garlic, pepper, smoked paprika, salt, and stevia. Mix until the ingredients are well incorporated. Form the mixture into four patties.

2. In a large sauté pan, heat the olive oil over medium-high heat until it shimmers. Add the bison patties to the pan, and cook without moving them until well browned, about 6 minutes per side.

3. Spread each of the hamburger buns with 1 tablespoon of Bistro Burger Sauce. Place a burger on each bun, and top with a tomato slice and some arugula.

REIGNITE

Dinner

Grilled Skirt Steak Chimichurri

SERVES 4 / PREP TIME: 10 MINUTES / COOK TIME: 6 MINUTES

Chimichurri sauce is a green herb and garlic sauce that hails from Argentina, where it's an essential accompaniment to grilled steak. It's also great on chicken and fish, as a marinade, and on vegetables.

Ingredient tip: *If you can't find skirt steak, you can substitute flank steak. To keep the steak tender, cut it across the grain before serving.*

1½ pounds skirt steak

Fine sea salt

Freshly ground black pepper

½ cup plus 2 tablespoons extra-virgin olive oil, divided

1 cup chopped fresh flat-leaf parsley

3 tablespoons chopped fresh oregano

3 garlic cloves, minced

⅓ cup red wine vinegar

Juice of 1 lime

¼ teaspoon red pepper flakes

1. Pound the skirt steak until it is an even thickness throughout. Season with salt and pepper, and let it sit for 20 minutes.

2. In a large sauté pan, heat 2 tablespoons olive oil over medium-high heat until it shimmers. Add the skirt steak, and cook without moving it until it sears on the bottom, 2 to 3 minutes. Flip the steak over, and cook it on the other side until it sears on the bottom, another 2 to 3 minutes.

3. Remove the steak from the pan, and allow it to rest on a platter, tented with foil to keep it warm, about 10 minutes.

4. While the steak rests, prepare the chimichurri sauce. In a blender or food processor, combine the remaining ½ cup olive oil, parsley, oregano, garlic, red wine vinegar, lime juice, and red pepper flakes. Process until the herbs are finely chopped, about 20 seconds.

5. Slice the skirt steak against the grain into ½-inch-thick strips. Serve with the chimichurri sauce spooned over the top.

Nut-free
Paleo-friendly

REIGNITE

Dinner

PER SERVING
CALORIES: 555
CARBS: 4G
FAT: 39G
PROTEIN: 46G
SUGAR: 0G

Minted Lamb Chops

SERVES 4 / PREP TIME: 15 MINUTES / COOK TIME: 10 MINUTES

Lamb and mint are a classic combination. In this recipe, mint and garlic balance the gamey flavors of the lamb, creating a delicious update on an old favorite. Trim the lamb chops of visible fat before cooking them. Serve these lamb chops with the Cannellini Bean Salad with Mint (page 253).

Technique tip: *You can also grill the lamb chops. Grill over medium-high direct heat until the lamb reaches an internal temperature of 145°F, about 5 minutes per side.*

Nut-free
Paleo-friendly

REIGNITE

Dinner

PER SERVING
CALORIES: 313
CARBS: 2G
FAT: 19G
PROTEIN: 32G
SUGAR: 0G

3 tablespoons olive oil

6 garlic cloves, minced

¼ cup chopped fresh mint

1 teaspoon ground cumin

½ teaspoon fine sea salt

½ teaspoon freshly ground black pepper

¼ teaspoon cayenne pepper

4 (4-ounce) lamb loin chops, trimmed

1. Preheat the broiler and place a rack in the middle of the oven.

2. In a blender or food processor, combine the olive oil, garlic, mint, cumin, salt, pepper, and cayenne. Process until the herbs are finely chopped.

3. Put the lamb chops on a broiler pan, and spread half the mint sauce over the top of the chops. Turn the chops over, and spread on the remaining sauce. Allow the lamb chops to sit, coated with the sauce, for 10 minutes.

4. Broil the lamb chops until they are browned, 4 to 5 minutes per side.

Mediterranean Spiced Lamb Burgers with Arugula Salad and Red Onion Quick Pickle

SERVES 4 / PREP TIME: 20 MINUTES, PLUS 2 HOURS TO CHILL /
COOK TIME: 15 MINUTES

Instead of a bun, this flavorful patty is served on a bed of peppery arugula. The red onion quick pickle and garlic mayonnaise vinaigrette add so much flavor that you won't even miss the bun. With olive oil in the vinaigrette, you'll also get plenty of healthy fats, along with protein in the burgers and fiber in the vegetables.

For the quick pickle

1 teaspoon sea salt

½ cup red wine vinegar

1 red onion, thinly sliced

For the burgers

1 pound ground lamb

4 garlic cloves, minced

1 teaspoon ground cumin

1 teaspoon ground coriander

1 teaspoon dried oregano

1 teaspoon sea salt

½ teaspoon freshly ground black pepper

For the salad

6 cups arugula

12 cherry tomatoes, halved

1 cucumber, chopped

4 tablespoons Easy Homemade Mayonnaise (page 37)

½ cup red wine vinegar

2 garlic cloves, passed through a garlic press

¼ teaspoon sea salt

½ teaspoon freshly ground black pepper »

Nut-free
Paleo-friendly

REIGNITE

Dinner

PER SERVING
CALORIES: 387
CARBS: 27G
FAT: 14G
PROTEIN: 37G
SUGAR: 14G

**Mediterranean Spiced Lamb Burgers with Arugula Salad and
Red Onion Quick Pickle** *continued*

To make the quick pickle

1. In a medium bowl, whisk together the salt and red wine vinegar until the salt dissolves.

2. Add the onion and push it to the bottom of the bowl, so it is submerged in the vinegar.

3. Cover and refrigerate for 2 hours.

To make the burgers

1. In a large bowl, combine the lamb, garlic, cumin, coriander, oregano, salt, and pepper. Mix with your hands until well combined. Form the mixture into four patties.

2. Heat a large nonstick pan over medium-high heat. Add the burgers, and cook until the lamb is 165°F in the center, about 6 or 7 minutes per side.

To make the salad

1. In a large bowl, combine the arugula, tomatoes, and cucumber. Toss to combine.

2. In a small bowl, whisk together the mayonnaise, red wine vinegar, garlic, salt, and pepper.

3. Pour the vinaigrette over the salad, and toss to combine.

4. To assemble, divide the salad among four plates. Top each salad with a burger patty. Top each burger with the quick pickled red onions.

Spiced Custard

SERVES 4 / PREP TIME: 20 MINUTES, PLUS 2 HOURS TO CHILL /
COOK TIME: 5 MINUTES

Vanilla and fall spices make these custards delicious. The custard is thickened with gelatin, which must soften in cold liquid before being dissolved in hot liquid. Therefore, the custard has a two-step process to make sure it sets correctly.

15 ounces light coconut milk

1 tablespoon gelatin

15 ounces full-fat coconut milk

1 teaspoon ground cinnamon

1 teaspoon ground ginger

½ teaspoon ground cloves

½ teaspoon ground nutmeg

Zest of ½ orange

Pinch of salt

3 packets stevia

1 teaspoon vanilla extract

Nut-free
Paleo-friendly
Vegetarian

REIGNITE

Dessert

PER SERVING
CALORIES: 186
CARBS: 7G
FAT: 18G
PROTEIN: 4G
SUGAR: 2G

1. In a small bowl, combine the light coconut milk and the gelatin. Set aside.

2. In a medium saucepan, combine the full-fat coconut milk, cinnamon, ginger, cloves, nutmeg, orange zest, salt, stevia, and vanilla. Heat the mixture over medium-high heat until it simmers.

3. Remove the pan from the heat, and whisk in the light coconut milk and gelatin.

4. Pour into four individual custard cups, and refrigerate for 2 hours, until the gelatin sets.

Vanilla Strawberries with Lemony Coconut Cream

SERVES 4 / PREP TIME: 20 MINUTES

In-season strawberries are the sweetest, so try to find strawberries from local farms during the peak summer season. Cold fruits sometimes have less flavor, so bring the strawberries to room temperature and taste them before adding sweetener.

1 tablespoon honey

2 teaspoons white balsamic vinegar

1 teaspoon vanilla extract

Pinch of fine sea salt

3 cups quartered strawberries

2 tablespoons freshly grated lemon zest

1 (15-ounce) can full-fat coconut milk

Nut-free
Paleo-friendly
Vegetarian

REIGNITE

Dessert

PER SERVING
CALORIES: 263
CARBS: 18G
FAT: 20G
PROTEIN: 3G
SUGAR: 11G

1. In a small bowl, whisk together the honey, white balsamic vinegar, vanilla, and salt until well combined. Add the strawberries, and stir to combine. Let stand at room temperature for at least 15 minutes, and up to 2 hours, stirring occasionally.

2. Just before serving, in another bowl, stir the lemon zest into the coconut milk.

3. Taste the strawberry mixture. If it's too tart, add a little more honey.

4. To serve, spoon ½ cup of the lemon-coconut milk into each of four dessert bowls, and top each with about ⅓ cup of the strawberries. Serve immediately.

Chocolate Strawberries

SERVES 4 / PREP TIME: 10 MINUTES / COOK TIME: 5 MINUTES

Choose extra-large, in-season strawberries for this decadent dessert. Extra-virgin coconut oil contains healthy fats and is solid at room temperature, so it's the perfect base for the chocolate coating. The strawberries will keep, tightly sealed, in the refrigerator for three days.

Time-saving tip: *If you're in a hurry, the chocolate will set very quickly if you refrigerate it right after dipping the strawberries. Place the berries on a parchment paper–lined tray and refrigerate for about 20 minutes.*

¼ cup unsweetened coconut flakes

¼ cup extra-virgin coconut oil

¾ cup chopped vegan dark chocolate

¼ teaspoon powdered stevia

12 strawberries

1. Line a baking sheet with parchment paper.

2. Spread out the coconut flakes in a shallow dish.

3. In a small saucepan, melt the coconut oil and chocolate over low heat, stirring constantly. Add the stevia. Taste and adjust the sweetener as needed. Remove from the heat.

4. Dip the strawberries in the chocolate, and then roll them in the coconut. Place them on the parchment-lined tray, and allow them to set at room temperature or in the refrigerator.

Nut-free
Paleo-friendly
Vegan

REIGNITE

Dessert

PER SERVING
CALORIES: 392
CARBS: 34G
FAT: 30G
PROTEIN: 4G
SUGAR: 2G

Chocolate-Dipped Blueberry Yogurt Bars

SERVES 4 / PREP TIME: 10 MINUTES, PLUS FREEZING TIME / COOK TIME: 5 MINUTES

You won't miss ice cream with these creamy bars. You need to make them in stages—freeze the bars first, and then coat them with chocolate. You can use ice pop molds for this recipe or paper cups and wooden sticks.

2 cups blueberries

2 cups plain, unsweetened almond milk yogurt or coconut milk yogurt

½ teaspoon powdered stevia, divided

¾ cup chopped vegan dark chocolate

¼ cup extra-virgin coconut oil

1 cup chopped toasted pecans

Paleo-friendly
Vegan

REIGNITE

Dessert

PER SERVING
CALORIES: 510
CARBS: 54G
FAT: 36G
PROTEIN: 4G
SUGAR: 15G

1. In a blender, combine the blueberries, yogurt, and ¼ teaspoon stevia. Blend on high speed until puréed.

2. Spoon the mixture into four small paper cups or ice pop molds. If using paper cups, cover the cups with foil and insert a wooden stick through the foil. Freeze overnight until solid.

3. When the ice pops are frozen, remove them from the molds (or peel away the paper cups) and place them on a tray in the freezer.

4. In a medium saucepan, melt the chocolate and coconut oil over low heat, stirring constantly. Stir in the remaining ¼ teaspoon stevia. Remove the chocolate from the heat and cool to room temperature.

5. Remove the ice pops from the freezer. Dip them in the chocolate mixture; then dip them in the chopped pecans. Wrap the ice pops in parchment paper, and freeze until the chocolate coating sets.

Chocolate Soufflés

SERVES 2 / PREP TIME: 15 MINUTES / COOK TIME: 25 MINUTES

These will not rise as much as regular soufflés, but they taste just as good. Serve them with Raspberry Sauce (page 211) or with any low-glycemic-index fruit, such as berries. Eat them while they are warm, topped with a dusting of unsweetened cocoa powder.

Ingredient tip: *When it comes to dark chocolate, the darker the better. Look for 85 percent cocoa (sometimes written 85 percent cacao), which means 85 percent of the contents of that product comes from cocoa beans. The higher the cocoa content, the greater the flavor intensity and the less added sugar.*

Nonstick cooking spray

2 teaspoons arrowroot powder, divided

2½ ounces vegan dark chocolate, chopped

1 egg yolk

1 tablespoon unsweetened, unflavored almond milk

¼ teaspoon powdered stevia

⅛ teaspoon ground cinnamon

3 egg whites

⅛ teaspoon fine sea salt

**Paleo-friendly
Vegetarian**

REIGNITE

Dessert

PER SERVING
CALORIES: 370
CARBS: 50G
FAT: 18G
PROTEIN: 11G
SUGAR: 7G

1. Preheat the oven to 375°F. Lightly coat two 10-ounce ramekins with nonstick cooking spray. Coat the inside of each with ½ teaspoon arrowroot powder.

2. In a double boiler over hot water, place the chocolate. Stir occasionally until it melts.

3. In a medium bowl, whisk together the egg yolk and almond milk until combined. Whisk in the chocolate until smooth; then whisk in the stevia, cinnamon, and remaining 1 teaspoon arrowroot powder.

4. In a medium bowl, beat the egg whites and salt with an electric mixer on high speed until soft peaks form.

5. Fold the chocolate mixture into the egg whites until smooth and even.

6. Divide between the prepared ramekins, and place on a baking sheet. Bake until firm to the touch, 18 to 22 minutes.

Chocolate-Peanut Butter Squares

MAKES 9 CANDIES / PREP TIME: 10 MINUTES / COOK TIME: 5 MINUTES

These sweet little chocolate squares are very simple to make, but they are so delicious. They will last for months in a zip-top bag in the refrigerator or freezer. You can replace the peanut butter with cashew butter or almond butter if you prefer.

½ cup extra-virgin coconut oil

½ cup unsweetened cocoa powder

3 tablespoons smooth peanut butter

¼ teaspoon powdered stevia

1. Line a 9-inch-square pan with parchment paper.

2. In a medium saucepan, heat the coconut oil, cocoa powder, and peanut butter over low heat until everything melts.

3. Stir in the stevia. Taste and adjust the sweetness.

4. Pour the mixture into the prepared pan. Refrigerate until the mixture sets.

5. Cut into 1-inch squares.

Vegan

REIGNITE

Dessert

PER SERVING
CALORIES: 153
CARBS: 4G
FAT: 16G
PROTEIN: 2G
SUGAR: 1G

Chocolate-Walnut Truffles

SERVES 8 / PREP TIME: 10 MINUTES, PLUS 1 HOUR CHILLING TIME

These crave-worthy chocolate-walnut truffles are creamy, sweet, and chocolatey. The almond butter and walnuts add beneficial fats, while the chocolate is rich in antioxidants and just plain delicious.

½ cup walnuts, chopped

½ cup almond butter

3 tablespoons unsweetened cocoa powder

3 packets stevia

½ cup unsweetened coconut flakes

1. In a small bowl, mix together the walnuts, almond butter, cocoa powder, and stevia.

2. Roll the mixture into eight balls.

3. Put the coconut on a plate. Roll the truffles in the coconut.

4. Refrigerate for 1 hour.

Paleo-friendly
Vegan

REIGNITE

Dessert

PER SERVING
CALORIES: 197
CARBS: 6G
FAT: 18G
PROTEIN: 6G
SUGAR: 1G

Macaroons

SERVES 12 / PREP TIME: 15 MINUTES / COOK TIME: 15 MINUTES

If you're craving a cookie, these macaroons will fit the bill. Rich with healthy coconut, these low-glycemic-index treats are very satisfying. They are the perfect bite for after dinner, offering a taste of something sweet without the sugar rush.

3 egg whites

¼ teaspoon ground cinnamon

2 packets stevia

1 tablespoon coconut oil, melted

½ teaspoon vanilla extract

Pinch of salt

1½ cups unsweetened shredded coconut

Nut-free
Paleo-friendly
Vegan

REIGNITE

Dessert

PER SERVING
CALORIES: 50
CARBS: 2G
FAT: 5G
PROTEIN: 1G
SUGAR: 1G

1. Preheat the oven to 350°F. Line a baking sheet with parchment paper.

2. In a medium bowl, use a hand mixer to beat the egg whites until they form soft peaks.

3. Stir in the cinnamon, stevia, coconut oil, vanilla, and salt.

4. Carefully fold the coconut into the mixture.

5. Drop in 12 spoonfuls onto the prepared baking sheet, leaving room between each cookie to spread.

6. Bake until the cookies turn golden around the edges, about 15 minutes.

7. Transfer to a wire rack and cool before serving.

Almond Butter Cookies

SERVES 12 / PREP TIME: 15 MINUTES / COOK TIME: 10 MINUTES

Almond butter has a lot going for it, including beneficial fats, iron, and loads of magnesium. It also makes a mighty delicious cookie. These cookies offer a hint of after-dinner sweetness without all the carbs, yet they are immensely satisfying. Enjoy them for a dessert or snack with a mug of light coconut milk, heated up and sprinkled with nutmeg.

Substitution tip: *You can replace the almond butter with your favorite unsweetened nut butter. Make sure the nut butter you use is sugar-free.*

1 egg, beaten
½ teaspoon almond extract
½ teaspoon vanilla extract
3 tablespoons honey
¼ cup coconut oil, melted
1 cup unsweetened almond butter
1¼ cups almond flour
½ teaspoon baking soda
1 packet stevia
½ teaspoon ground cinnamon
¼ teaspoon ground nutmeg
Dash of sea salt

Paleo-friendly
Vegetarian

REIGNITE

Dessert

PER SERVING
CALORIES: 211
CARBS: 9G
FAT: 18G
PROTEIN: 6G
SUGAR: 5G

1. Preheat the oven to 350°F. Line a baking sheet with parchment paper.

2. In a small bowl, whisk together the egg, almond extract, vanilla, honey, and coconut oil until well combined. Whisk in the almond butter.

3. In a large bowl, whisk together the almond flour, baking soda, stevia, cinnamon, nutmeg, and salt.

4. Pour the egg mixture into the almond flour mixture. Stir until well mixed.

5. Drop the dough by tablespoonfuls onto the prepared baking sheet, leaving room for the cookies to spread.

6. Bake until the cookies brown around the edges, about 8 minutes.

7. Cool on a wire rack before serving.

APPENDIX A:

A Sample 28-Day Meal Plan

This sample 28-day meal plan offers suggestions for every breakfast, lunch, dinner, snack, and dessert for your 28 days on the Fast Metabolism Diet. Use this as your guide as you work your way through the recipes in this book. We've included dessert suggestions for every day, but you're only required to eat five meals a day. If you're craving something sweet, have a dessert and one snack rather than two snacks. Or have all six meals, and add one more day of stage-appropriate exercise to your week.

Week One

*An asterisk denotes recipes in this book.

Monday: Repair
Breakfast: Blueberry-Banana Smoothie*
Snack: 1 green apple
Lunch: Gazpacho*
Snack: 1 banana
Dinner: Shrimp with Tropical Fruit Salsa* and steamed broccoli
Dessert: Cantaloupe Seed Drink*

Tuesday: Repair
Breakfast: Almond Butter and Banana Toast*
Snack: Herbal Tea Smoothie*
Lunch: Gingered Peach and Rice Salad*
Snack: 1 nectarine
Dinner: Black Bean Soup with Ground Turkey and Sweet Potatoes*
Dessert: Fruit Medley*

Wednesday: Release
Breakfast: Breakfast Tacos*
Snack: Jicama Sticks with Chili and Lime*
Lunch: Gingered Chicken Salad*
Snack: 2 slices deli roast beef
Dinner: Spinach-Stuffed Fillet of Sole with Green Beans*
Dessert: Cranberry-Orange Compote*

Thursday: Release
Breakfast: Fresh Veggie Frittata*
Snack: 2 celery ribs
Lunch: Gingered Chicken Salad*
Snack: Lemony Tuna and Radishes*
Dinner: Turkey Lettuce Cups*
Dessert: Chocolate Pudding*

Friday: Reignite
Breakfast: Fruit and Greens Smoothie*
Snack: 2 hardboiled eggs
Lunch: Tuna Salad*
Snack: 2 celery ribs with 2 tablespoons almond butter
Dinner: Carrot-Ginger Soup with Kale Pesto*
Dessert: Sliced strawberries

Saturday: Reignite
Breakfast: Pumpkin Pancakes*
Snack: Grapes
Lunch: Pork Tenderloin with Mustard and Plums*
Snack: Pumpkin Dip*
Dinner: Cioppino*
Dessert: Kiwi-Strawberry Ice Pops*

Sunday: Reignite
Breakfast: Hot Quinoa Breakfast Cereal with Flax*
Lunch: Easy Chicken Rice Soup*
Snack: Pumpkin Dip*
Dinner: Orange Beef Stir-Fry* and cauliflower rice (see Slow Cooker Red Pepper
    Stuffed with Italian Ground Turkey and Cauliflower, page 160)
Dessert: Watermelon
Snack: Banana

Week Two

*An asterisk denotes recipes in this book.

Monday: Repair
Breakfast: Green Tea Smoothie*
Snack: 1 orange
Lunch: Minted Cantaloupe and Cucumber Salad*
Snack: Black Bean and Pineapple Salsa with Corn Chips*
Dinner: Cowboy Steak with Grilled Peaches*
Dessert: Honeydew and Berries*

Tuesday: Repair
Breakfast: Breakfast Rice*
Snack: 1 nectarine
Lunch: Open-Faced Prosciutto, Fig, and Arugula Sandwich*
Snack: Mediterranean White Bean Dip with Vegetables*
Dinner: Pork with Fava Beans and Strawberries*
Dessert: Tea-Steeped Plums*

Wednesday: Release
Breakfast: Scrambled egg whites and mushrooms
Snack: 2 slices deli roast beef
Lunch: Meatballs with Spinach*
Snack: 8 baby carrots
Dinner: Vegetable Soup with Clams and Greens*
Dessert: Hot Chocolate*

Thursday: Release
Breakfast: Salmon Scramble*
Snack: 2 slices deli roast beef
Lunch: Roast Beef Roll-Ups*
Snack: 1 hardboiled egg
Dinner: Roasted Portobello Mushrooms with Garlic-Cauliflower Mash*
Dessert: Cranberry-Orange Compote*

Friday: Reignite
Breakfast: Scrambled Eggs Florentine*
Snack: Jicama sticks and jarred salsa
Lunch: Chicken Caesar Salad with Cashews*
Snack: Cantaloupe and Prosciutto*
Dinner: Grilled Skirt Steak Chimichurri* and steamed asparagus
Dessert: Chocolate-Dipped Blueberry Yogurt Bars*

Saturday: Reignite
Breakfast: Tex-Mex Eggs with Black Beans and Avocados*
Snack: Cantaloupe wedges
Lunch: Ham and Egg Salad Sandwich*
Snack: Cannellini Bean Salad with Mint*
Dinner: Chicken Satay with Peanut Sauce* and tossed salad with oil and vinegar
Dessert: Chocolate-Peanut Butter Squares*

Sunday: Reignite
Breakfast: Vegetable and Egg Baked Breakfast*
Snack: Jicama sticks with jarred salsa
Lunch: Tuna Salad*
Snack: Cantaloupe wedges
Dinner: Calamari Salad*
Dessert: Chocolate-Peanut Butter Squares*

Week Three

*An asterisk denotes recipes in this book.

Monday: Repair

Breakfast: Spiced Baked Apples with Flax*
Snack: 1 orange
Lunch: Tomato and Orange Chopped Salad*
Snack: Mediterranean White Bean Dip with Vegetables*
Dinner: Rack of Lamb with Apricot Relish*
Dessert: Kiwi-Strawberry Ice Pops*

Tuesday: Repair

Breakfast: Pumpkin Pancakes*
Snack: Grapes
Lunch: Pork Tenderloin with Mustard and Plums*
Snack: Pumpkin Dip*
Dinner: Cioppino*
Dessert: Kiwi-Strawberry Ice Pops*

Wednesday: Release

Breakfast: Turkey Breakfast Sausage* and scrambled egg whites
Snack: Salmon Cucumber Rounds*
Lunch: Slow Cooker Chicken Thighs with Cauliflower and Carrot Salad*
Snack: 2 slices deli roast beef
Dinner: Pork Chops with Mushrooms*
Dessert: Chocolate Pudding*

Thursday: Release

Breakfast: Sausage, Egg White, and Kale Breakfast Skillet*
Snack: 8 baby carrots
Lunch: Chicken Fajitas*
Snack: Smoked Trout Wraps*
Dinner: Halibut Niçoise*
Dessert: Lemon Granita* with Raspberry Sauce*

Friday: Reignite

Breakfast: Tex-Mex Eggs with Black Beans and Avocados*
Snack: Sliced apple with 2 tablespoons almond butter
Lunch: Ginger Chicken Slaw*
Snack: Red Pepper Hummus with Crudités*
Dinner: Baked Cod with Tomatoes, Asparagus, and Olives*
Dessert: Chocolate-Dipped Blueberry Yogurt Bars*

Saturday: Reignite

Breakfast: Scrambled eggs with ½ sliced avocado
Snack: Apple slices with 2 tablespoons almond butter
Lunch: Crab Cakes with Sriracha Mayonnaise*
Snack: Red Pepper Hummus with Crudités*
Dinner: Three-Bean Chili*
Dessert: Chocolate Strawberries*

Sunday: Reignite

Breakfast: Canadian Bacon and Bell Pepper Omelet*
Snack: Celery with 2 tablespoons almond butter
Lunch: Chicken Salad with Broccoli and Tomatoes*
Snack: Roasted Eggplant Spread*
Dinner: Macadamia-Crusted Halibut*
Dessert: Chocolate-Dipped Blueberry Yogurt Bars*

Week Four

*An asterisk denotes recipes in this book.

Monday: Repair

Breakfast: Almond Butter and Banana Toast*
Snack: 1 green apple
Lunch: Open-Faced Prosciutto, Fig, and Arugula Sandwich*
Snack: Herbal Tea Smoothie*
Dinner: Baked Scallops with Mango Salsa*
Dessert: Honeydew and Berries*

Tuesday: Repair

Breakfast: Blueberry-Banana Smoothie*
Snack: Black Bean and Pineapple Salsa with Corn Chips*
Lunch: Easy Chicken Rice Soup*
Snack: 1 green apple
Dinner: Orange Beef Stir-Fry* and rice
Dessert: Cantaloupe Seed Drink*

Wednesday: Release

Breakfast: Salmon Scramble*
Snack: Jicama Sticks with Chili and Lime*
Lunch: Roast Beef Roll-Ups*
Snack: 2 slices deli ham
Dinner: Lemony Mussels with Green Beans, Fennel, and Red Bell Pepper*
Dessert: Hot Chocolate*

Thursday: Release

Breakfast: Fresh Veggie Frittata*
Snack: 2 slices deli ham
Lunch: Gingered Chicken Salad*
Snack: Salmon Cucumber Rounds*
Dinner: Poached Chicken and Mixed Vegetables*
Dessert: Lemon Granita*

Friday: Reignite

Breakfast: Fruit and Greens Smoothie*
Snack: Apple slices with 2 tablespoons almond butter
Lunch: Tuna Salad*
Snack: Cantaloupe and Prosciutto*
Dinner: Shrimp with Summer Squash*
Dessert: Chocolate Strawberries*

Saturday: Reignite

Breakfast: Scrambled Eggs Florentine*
Snack: Celery with 2 tablespoons almond butter
Lunch: Ham and Egg Salad Sandwich*
Snack: Red Pepper Hummus with Crudités*
Dinner: Veal Piccata* and steamed broccoli
Dessert: Chocolate-Dipped Blueberry Yogurt Bars*

Sunday: Reignite

Breakfast: Steel-Cut Oats with Walnuts and Spices*
Snack: Sliced cantaloupe
Lunch: Crab Cakes with Sriracha Mayonnaise*
Snack: Fruit and Fennel Yogurt*
Dinner: Minted Lamb Chops*
Dessert: Chocolate Strawberries*

Tips for Eating Out

Who wants to cook all the time? Going to restaurants and enjoying meals with friends and family is an important part of socializing. However, anyone who has ever tried to eat out while following a diet knows how difficult it can be. Restaurants offer dishes that sabotage your best efforts with a single bite.

The secret to eating out and staying on the Fast Metabolism Diet is to be prepared before you arrive at the restaurant. Here are some tips and suggestions to help you resist unhealthy temptations:

Plan Ahead. Go online and see what the restaurant has to offer that you can eat. If there's grilled fish, chicken, or shrimp on the menu, you'll know that you have several choices.

Order Differently. Many restaurants have a wealth of healthy eating choices—if you know what to order.

- **Mexican:** Refuse the basket of tortilla chips. Perhaps you can order some cut-up vegetables to go with the salsa instead. Fajitas made with grilled beef, chicken, shrimp, or vegetables and piled with lettuce, diced tomatoes, and onions make a great low-fat choice. Beans and rice are good, but hold the cheese, sour cream, and tortillas.

- **Italian:** Select salad or a half order of pasta with light tomato sauce, red clam sauce, or shrimp marinara. Avoid cream-based sauces. For other entrées, order chicken cacciatore, chicken piccata sautéed in olive oil, shrimp scampi cooked in olive oil, or grilled fish.

- **Chinese:** Opt for steamed or stir-fried seafood, chicken, or vegetables dishes with steamed rice. And don't forget to ask the chef to go easy on the oil and soy sauce. Skip fried egg rolls and wontons, stir-fried noodles, General Tso's chicken, sweet and sour pork, and fried rice. All of those dishes are prepared with lots of oil and sodium.

Don't Arrive Hungry. If you sit down starving, your eyes will go straight for the big-portion, high-carb, high-fat selections on the menu. Eat a low-fat snack beforehand, such as yogurt, nuts, and fruit. It will protect you from eyeing unhealthy selections.

Watch the Menu Words: Many menus nowadays highlight healthy or low-fat dishes or alternatives. Choose items that are grilled, broiled, poached, or steamed, and ask your waiter to omit any sauces from your order. Anything that is creamed, buttered, fried, crispy, or breaded should be avoided. If you're not sure, ask the waiter for details.

Order a Salad First. Studies show that people who eat salads before or with their meals tend to eat less food. A big salad full of crunchy vegetables is a perfect meal. Make sure to stick with healthy oil and vinegar instead of dressings like ranch, Thousand Island, and honey mustard, which are often high in fat and calories.

Soup Up: Order a low-calorie vegetable soup before your entrée. People who eat soup before their main meal can reduce their total dinner calorie intake by 20 percent, according to a study from Penn State University. Avoid cream-based soups and those topped with cheese or croutons.

Keep Drinking Water. Fill up your water glass through your meal. It will help keep your appetite in check and stop you from reaching for seconds and thirds.

Half Is Better Than Full: Restaurants are famous for huge, oversized portions. Ask if someone wants to share an entrée with you. Or ask that your entrée be served with a to-go container, and place half of your portion into it before eating. If it's off your plate, you won't be tempted to eat it.

The Dirty Dozen and the Clean Fifteen

Each year, the Environmental Working Group (EWG), an environmental organization based in the United States, publishes a list they call "The Dirty Dozen." These are the fruits and vegetables that, when conventionally grown using chemical pesticides and fertilizers, carry the highest residues. If organically grown isn't an option for you, simply avoid these fruits and vegetables altogether. The list is updated each year, but here is the most recent list (2014).

Similarly, the EWG publishes a list of "The Clean Fifteen," fruits and vegetables that, even when conventionally grown, contain very low levels of chemical pesticide or fertilizer residue. These items are acceptable to purchase conventionally grown. You might want to snap a photo of these two lists and keep them on your phone to reference while shopping. Or you can download the EWG's app to your phone or tablet.

The Dirty Dozen	The Clean Fifteen
Apples	Asparagus
Bell peppers	Avocados
Celery	Cabbage
Cherry tomatoes	Cantaloupe
Cucumbers	Corn
Grapes	Eggplant
Nectarines (imported)	Grapefruit
Peaches	Kiwi
Potatoes	Mangos
Snap peas	Mushrooms
Spinach	Onions
Strawberries	Papayas
	Pineapples
	Sweet peas (frozen)
	Sweet potatoes

Measurement Conversions

Volume Equivalents (Liquid)

US STANDARD	US STANDARD (OUNCES)	METRIC (APPROXIMATE)
2 tablespoons	1 fl. oz.	30 mL
¼ cup	2 fl. oz.	60 mL
½ cup	4 fl. oz.	120 mL
1 cup	8 fl. oz.	240 mL
1½ cups	12 fl. oz.	355 mL
2 cups or 1 pint	16 fl. oz.	475 mL
4 cups or 1 quart	32 fl. oz.	1 L
1 gallon	128 fl. oz.	4 L

Oven Temperatures

FAHRENHEIT (F)	CELSIUS (C) (APPROXIMATE)
250	120
300	150
325	165
350	180
375	190
400	200
425	220
450	230

Volume Equivalents (Dry)

US STANDARD	METRIC (APPROXIMATE)
⅛ teaspoon	.05 mL
¼ teaspoon	1 mL
½ teaspoon	2 mL
¾ teaspoon	4 mL
1 teaspoon	5 mL
1 tablespoon	15 mL
¼ cup	59 mL
⅓ cup	79 mL
½ cup	118 mL
⅔ cup	156 mL
¾ cup	177 mL
1 cup	235 mL
2 cups or 1 pint	475 mL
3 cups	700 mL
4 cups or 1 quart	1 L
½ gallon	2 L
1 gallon	4 L

Weight Equivalents

US STANDARD	METRIC (APPROXIMATE)
½ ounce	15 g
1 ounce	30 g
2 ounces	60 g
4 ounces	115 g
8 ounces	225 g
12 ounces	340 g
16 ounces or 1 pound	455 g

Resources

Books

Here are some other titles related to the Fast Metabolism Diet you may find helpful:

Harriss, Helen. *Fast Metabolism Diet Recipes Under 30 Minutes: 74 Mouth-Watering Recipes for Breakfast, Lunch, Dinner, and Snacks.* Seattle: Bright Eye Press, 2014.

Hyman, Mark. *Ultrametabolism: The Simple Plan for Automatic Weight Loss.* New York: Atria Books, 2006.

Kress, Diane. *The Metabolism Miracle: Three Easy Steps to Regain Control of Your Weight . . . Permanently.* Philadelphia: Da Capo Books, 2009.

Marcum, Angela. *Fast Metabolism Diet Cookbook: Healthy, Wholesome, and Delectable Fast Metabolism Diet Recipes to Slim Down and Burn Fat.* Seattle: GMP Press, 2013.

Michaels, Jillian. *Master Your Metabolism.* New York: Three Rivers Press, 2009.

Mosley, Michael, and Mimi Spencer. *The Fast Diet: Lose Weight, Stay Healthy, and Live Longer with the Simple Secret of Intermittent Fasting.* New York: Atria Books, 2013.

New Health CookBooks. *My Fast Metabolism Diet Cookbook: The Wheat-Free, Soy-Free, Dairy-Free, Corn-Free, and Sugar-Free Cookbook.* Seattle: CreateSpace, 2013.

Pomroy, Haylie, and Eve Adamson. *The Fast Metabolism Diet: Eat More Food & Lose More Weight.* New York: Harmony Books, 2013.

Websites

Looking for medical information on how metabolism works and its link to weight loss? Check out these sites:

Increase Your Metabolism
www.webmd.com/diet/features/
increase-your-metabolism-start-losing-fat

Make the Most of Your Metabolism
www.webmd.com/diet/features/make-most
-your-metabolism

How to Lose Weight and Save Money
www.healthline.com/health-blogs/fitness
-fixer/metabolism-how-lose-weight-and-
save-money

How You Burn Calories
www.mayoclinic.org/healthy-living
weight-loss/in-depth/metabolism/
art-20046508

Weight-Loss Tools

Find your basal metabolic rate (BMR)—the number of calories your burn at rest.

www.myfitnesspal.com/tools/
bmr-calculator

Use this body calculator to find out your BMI, healthy weight range, daily calorie target, and more:

www.webmd.com/diet/healthtool -metabolism-calculator

Haylie Pomroy, author of *The Fast Metabolism Diet*, has an app that includes menu planning, food lists, grocery lists, and a tracker. The Fast Metabolism Diet App is available for iPhone and iPad at https:// itunes.apple.com.

References

Andrade, Ana M., MD, Geoffrey W. Greene, PhD, RD, and Kathleen J. Melanson, PhD, RD. "Eating Slowly Led to Decreases in Energy Intake within Meals in Healthy Women" in *Journal of the American Dietetic Association*. Volume 108, Issue 7 (July 2008).

Colorado State University Extension. "Nutrition and Aging." Accessed October 29, 2014. www.ext.colostate.edu/pubs/foodnut/09322.html

Mann, Denise. "Sleep and Weight Gain." Sleep Disorders Health Center, WebMD. Accessed October 29, 2014. www.webmd.com/sleep-disorders/excessive-sleepiness-10/lack-of-sleep-weight-gain

Pomroy, Haylie, and Eve Adamson. *The Fast Metabolism Diet: Eat More Food & Lose More Weight.* New York: Harmony Books, 2013.

Seematter, G., C. Binnert, and L. Tappy. "Stress and Metabolism." *Metabolic Syndrome and Related Disorders* 3, no. 1 (2005): 8–13. doi: 10.1089/met.2005.3.8.

Taubes, Gary. *Good Calories, Bad Calories: Challenging the Conventional Wisdom on Diet, Weight Control, and Disease.* New York: Knopf, 2007.

Index

B

Baba ghanoush, 259
Bacon. *See* Canadian bacon; Turkey bacon
Baked Cod with Tomatoes, Asparagus, and Olives, 279–280
Baked Red Snapper with Summer Fruit, 99
Baked Scallops with Mango Salsa, 104
Baked Scotch Eggs with Spinach, 146
Baked Sweet Potato Crisps, 82
Baked Sweet Potato with Pineapple, 97
Baking pans, 41
Baking sheet, 41
Bananas
    Almond Butter and Banana Toast, 57
    Blueberry-Banana Smoothie, 49
    Chocolate Shake, 79
    Fruit Medley, 125
    Green Tea Smoothie, 50
    Shrimp with Tropical Fruit Salsa, 105
Basil
    Baked Red Snapper with Summer Fruit, 99
    Breakfast Trout with Herbs and Eggs, 138–139
    Canadian Bacon and Kale Pesto Roll-Ups, 141
    Cobb Salad with Shrimp, 240
    Crispy Toasts with Tomato Basil Bruschetta, 87
    Gazpacho, 69
    Ham, Basil, and Spinach Rolls, 180
    Italian Chopped Salad with Ham, Tomatoes, and Peppers, 247
    Macadamia-Crusted Halibut, 281

Meatballs with Spinach, 166
Scrambled Eggs Florentine, 228
Slow Cooker Red Pepper Stuffed with Italian Ground Turkey and Cauliflower, 160–161
Spinach Salad with Chicken and Pesto Vinaigrette, 157
Zucchini Noodles with Meat Sauce, 203–204
BBQ Baked Beans and Greens, 94–95
Beans. *See* Black beans; Cannellini beans; Chickpeas; Kidney beans; Navy beans; Pinto beans
Beef, 33. *See also* Ground beef
    Beef with Broccoli, 209–210
    Cowboy Steak with Grilled Peaches, 119
    Grilled Skirt Steak Chimichurri, 295
    Orange Beef Stir-Fry, 118
    Roast Beef Roll-Ups, 167
Beefsteak tomatoes
    Black Bean Burger Wraps, 269–270
    Chef's Salad, 286
    Ham and Egg Salad Sandwich, 248
    Salmon Scramble, 140
    Tex-Mex Eggs with Black Beans and Avocados, 231
    Tomato and Orange Chopped Salad, 65
    Tuna Salad, 243
    Turkey Taco Salad, 158–159
    Vegetable and Egg Baked Breakfast, 229
Bell peppers, 34. *See also* Green bell peppers; Red bell peppers; Yellow bell peppers
Berries, 34. *See also* Blackberries; Blueberries; Cranberries; Raspberries; Strawberries

Beverages. *See also* Shakes; Smoothies
    Cantaloupe Seed Drink, 120
    Hot Chocolate, 218
Bibb lettuce
    Halibut Niçoise, 195–196
    Smoked Trout Wraps, 178
    Tuna Salad, 243
Bison Burgers with Bistro Burger Sauce, 293–294
Black beans, 36
    Black Bean and Pineapple Salsa with Corn Chips, 85
    Black Bean Burger Wraps, 269–270
    Black Bean Soup with Ground Turkey and Sweet Potatoes, 106
    Root Vegetables with Zesty Black Bean Dip, 258
    Tex-Mex Eggs with Black Beans and Avocados, 231
    Three-Bean Chili, 267–268
Blackberries
    Blackberry-Pomegranate Salad, 126
    Chicken Breasts with Blackberry Sauce, 75
    French Toast with Warm Berry Compote, 61–62
Black peppercorns, 39
Blenders, 40
Blood glucose, 17
Blood sugar, 18
Blueberry-Banana Smoothie, 49
Blueberries
    Almond Flour Pancakes with Orange-Blueberry Topping, 226–227
    Baked Red Snapper with Summer Fruit, 99
    Blueberries with Coconut Cream, 215
    Blueberry-Banana Smoothie, 49
    Chocolate-Dipped Blueberry Yogurt Bars, 302

CPSIA information can be obtained
at www.ICGtesting.com
Printed in the USA
LVIIW060835110319
609786LV00034B/121/P